# Hands and Heart

# Hands and Heart
## Stories of General Surgery

Michael DeHaan, MD

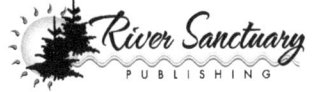

HANDS AND HEART

Copyright © 2013 by Michael DeHaan MD

All rights reserved. No part of this book may be reproduced in any form or by any electronic or mechanical means including information storage and retrieval systems, without permission in writing from the author. The only exception is by a reviewer, who may quote short excerpts in a review.

ISBN 978-1-935914-29-7

Cover and interior design by River Sanctuary Graphic Arts

Printed in the United States of America

To order additional copies please visit:
**www.riversanctuarypublishing.com**

Library of Congress Control Number: 2013946196

Send comments to:
handsandheart59@gmail.com

River Sanctuary Publishing
P.O Box 1561
Felton, CA 95018
**www.riversanctuarypublishing.com**

*Dedicated to the awakening of the New Earth*

*To my wife Barb*
*who has opened my mind*
*to a deeper experience of life*

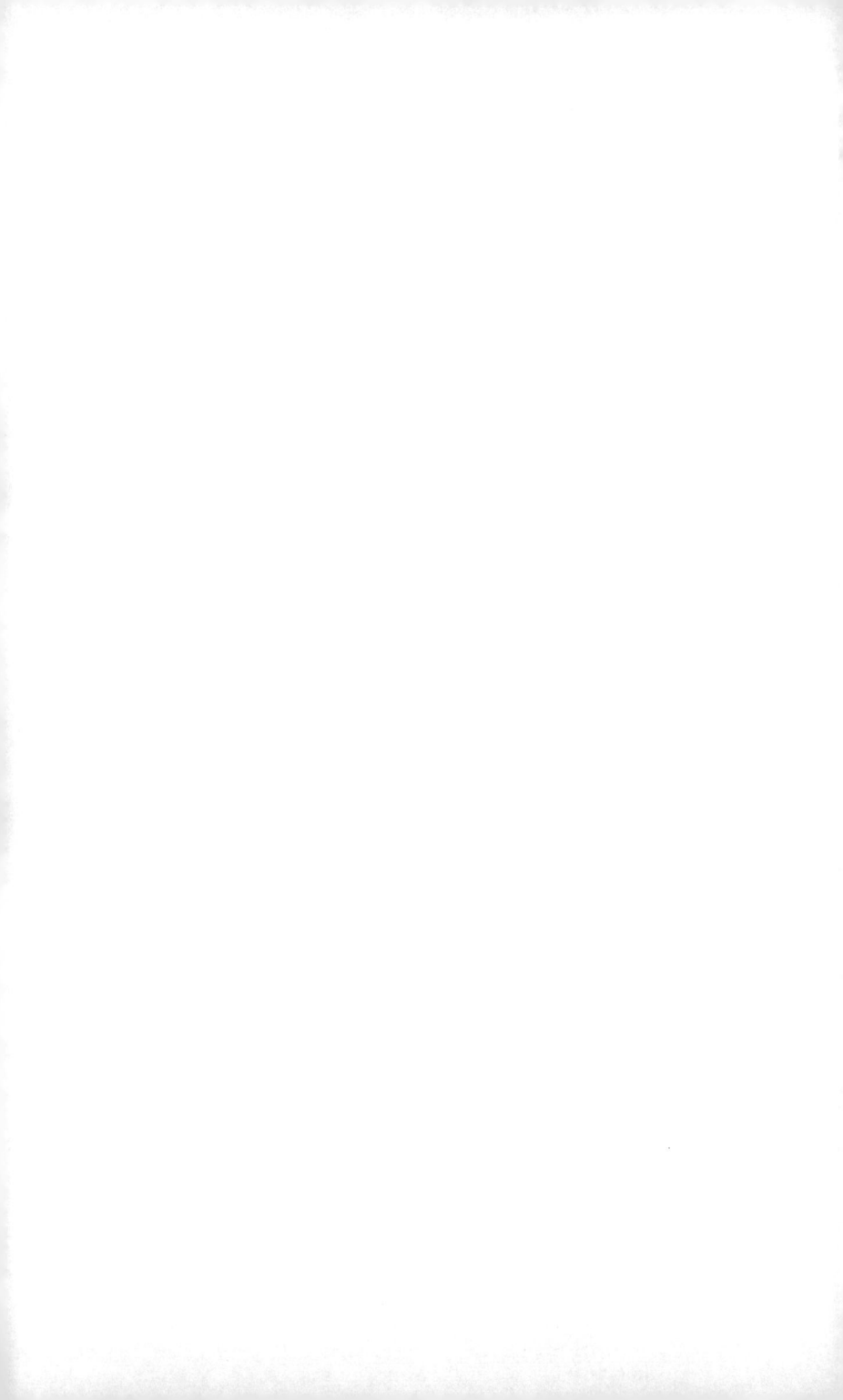

# Contents

Introduction .................................................... 1
The Heart of a Surgeon .................................... 3
Looking for the Dead Woman ......................... 7
Lessons in Survival .......................................... 9
Stress Tolls ..................................................... 13
Wooden Shoe Saves the Day ......................... 16
Attitude Adjustment ...................................... 19
Guatemala Adventure ................................... 22
A Day at the Office ........................................ 25
Blood and Blindness ..................................... 27
Eat a Big Breakfast ........................................ 30
Karma ............................................................ 32
Bad Day ......................................................... 34
Jake the Motorcycle Man .............................. 37
Life on Call .................................................... 38
Fun Yet? ......................................................... 41
Midnight Bleeder .......................................... 44
Two Whipples ............................................... 47
Symptoms and Outcomes ............................. 49
Making a Difference ..................................... 52
Surgery Isn't Hard To Do .............................. 55
King James Day ............................................. 58
The Fight for Life .......................................... 60
The Long Week ............................................. 63
Hit the Road .................................................. 67
The Assistant's Down .................................... 69
Just Checking… ............................................. 71
Not Social Anymore ..................................... 74
The Long Road to Life .................................. 76
The Other Side of Pain ................................. 78

| | |
|---|---|
| Call Again | 80 |
| No Vitals | 83 |
| Margaritaville and the Mudder Horse | 84 |
| Joy of Surgery | 88 |
| Expert help | 91 |
| Falling Scalpel | 93 |
| Appendix Once and for All | 95 |
| Incidental Miracles | 97 |
| Hits and Heroics | 100 |
| Not tonight, Frank | 105 |
| Epilogue | 107 |

# Introduction

My dad had owned a hardware store, then a business building houses. I grew up in that environment and imagined that I would eventually follow in his footsteps. Then my dad changed his direction and dedicated himself to full time Christian work.

When I went to college, I signed up for business and pre-seminary (reflecting my dad's orientation to life!?!). In my final choice to become a surgeon, I probably landed somewhere in between.

The path to surgery entails four years of regular college, four years of medical school, five to six years of "residency," or surgery training—after which one is at long last eligible to practice surgery. I entered my career as a surgeon at age 32, which is typical.

These are my stories, although one of them, as noted, was passed on to me. Others are too personal and can't be told. Many of them came to me in the middle of the night or the early hours of the morning. When this occurred, I would jot down a rough outline until such time as I could fill in the entire text, the words seeming to "spill out onto the page." The essence of each story is as true to fact as I can remember it. Of course, the names have been changed.

The winding road of the practice of surgery continues to fascinate me. Some stories point to the courage of the patient (or doctor!). Some celebrate the fascination of the medicine or the human body. Some are a reflection of how crazy it can get. My hope is that the reader, through these glimpses into the tapestry that is general surgery, will come away with an appreciation of the underlying human experience that touches us all.

*Surgeons heal with steel.*

# The Heart of a Surgeon

"I don't really think I need that big IV," the patient, Lyle, told me.

"You don't understand. This is required," I answered. He looked puzzled, but gave in.

His appearance was that of a distinguished, late middle-aged executive. I was on surgery service with the head of our program, and things could get a little wild. No matter what, my job required that I have the IV in this patient…

\*\*\*\*\*

Surgical residency had its moments.

The head of our program loved to "add on" cases in the middle of the night (adding a surgery case to the operating schedule for the following day). So at 2:00 AM a case might suddenly show up on the work docket for the next day. The fact that he decided to add it on late did not release us from the expectation that it would be our job to accumulate all the information by the morning. Tired and challenged, I don't think any of us appreciated it at the time. Looking back, I understand it was a game designed to teach us.

One night, after a particularly late "add on," we talked hospital security into letting us into his office. We rifled through his desk, found the x-ray films and reports, and took them. We then called the radiologist and pathologist at home (in the middle of the night) and arranged for them to come in early to read the x-rays and pathology so we could have a typed report on time in the morning.

The director came down as scheduled at 7:15 AM. He appeared ready to let us have it. I expect he believed he could catch us off guard by putting the case on the schedule at such an odd hour. Fortunately we had made friends with the nursing supervisor, who had clued us in to the schedule change. I stood at the x-ray board with all the information posted. He looked, speechless, and left without saying a word. We dodged that bullet.

I remember him stepping over a resident who had fainted. The resident had been up all night and hadn't had anything to eat. He stepped over the collapsed resident so he could position himself in the OR (operating room). He asked for another resident to be brought in right away to fill the vacant spot at the OR table. I assumed this came from a belief on his part that you have to be tough to do surgery. Perhaps he was right in this regard. We were left to pick the guy up and take care of him without interfering with the progress of the case.

One day we had a photo op. The director (Chief of Surgery) needed pictures of himself for something or other. The available case was a hernia, but he wanted us to make it look like a laser liver resection. We doubled the usual staff around the table, turned off the lights (except for the directed OR lights) and donned laser goggles. It made a fairly dramatic presentation. Pictures were taken.

The Chief of Surgery then did a portion of the hernia repair. He didn't do hernia repairs very often anymore. Eventually he left for a corner of the room to take more pictures in front of the x-ray light board. The chief resident/senior resident recognized that the repair was not up to standard, so while the director had his pictures taken, my chief resident made me take out the stitches and redo the hernia. I was a little concerned about getting caught doing that. Overall, however, it struck me as interesting that we were redoing his hernia at the same exact time he was posing for his pictures.

*****

So I took my executive man friend patient Lyle into surgery. He still looked puzzled. "You know, this isn't a very big surgery."

"I have my requirements," I told him.

We prepared things. My director came down and was ready to get going. We had a new nurse and somehow she had been left briefly on her own. The director/surgeon asked for a drape. She handed him the wrong one. He flung it like a frisbee, clearing off a fair amount of the back table instruments and supplies. Glass was flying and breaking. A lot of scrambling started. The regular nurse came running in and calmed things down.

Meanwhile, I caught a glance from the patient, who now seemed to understand a little better why I was careful about doing my job exactly as I was supposed to.

So we got going.

The director gave about 1 ml of numbing injection (essentially a few drops). Typically, today, I would give 10 to 20 mL to accomplish the same job and then check if the numbing "had taken." He started operating. From behind the drape I heard grunting and a little wiggling. I gently noted, "I'm not sure he's numb."

My director asked tersely, "Are you having pain?"

"Uh..uh..uh...no." We finished up. The patient didn't say anything more. I don't think he ever became numb, because I heard muffled noises and saw a little wiggling until we finished. When it was all over, I received a sympathetic nod from my patient.

*****

What is most striking to me is that in some sideways fashion, we didn't consider any of this unusual. Not in terms of the craziness of the story, but in terms of the impact it had on us personally. I think in the end, we had the bug for surgery. So often, medical students coming through the surgery rotation remarked about how much they loved surgery. It was understandable. It really is amazing. In some subtle way, I think we understood how amazing it was. In the same strange way, our desire to do it was in proportion to the fascination we had for the work. I can't tell you how often I've seen people "get the bug" and put up with almost anything to get the chance to do surgery.

People come to me and say "I could've been a surgeon." Sometimes it's one of my friends or family. Once in a while they'll hold up their hands and show me how steady they are. (I don't tell them that I can easily steady myself by resting my wrist on the table). Other times it's a colleague or doctor in training. While dexterity may count some, I think what really makes a surgeon is the heart. The wins can be big. The losses can be big too. You have to have enough self-confidence to believe that you did the right thing, or your first big loss will take you out permanently. But you can't have so much ego that you never question or look back or reoperate when something doesn't seem right.

I have a theory that we physicians are paid in proportion to our ability to have someone die under our care. A neurosurgeon works in an atmosphere where instantaneous death is possible if unforeseen circumstances arise. If the heart gets into trouble during cardiac surgery, it probably takes about five minutes to lose a patient. In general surgery, oftentimes it's a week or two of infection and difficulties before someone will die. With treatment of diabetes or hypertension, it could be years before the effects play out. Typically, this would also list them in decreasing order of pay. This also may partly get at the "heart" that it takes to do each of these jobs, related somehow to the "heat in the kitchen."

> Bard-Parker is a manufacturer of scalpels. A "Bard-Parker Scan" is opening the abdomen with a large incision to figure out the diagnosis when all other scans and biopsies have failed (a true "exploratory laparotomy").

## Looking for the Dead Woman

Anneka was as nice as could be, but very heavy. She had an abscess in the pelvis from diverticulitis. One of the little pockets off the side of her colon had become infected and ruptured. They had drained it with a needle and a tube in the CT scanner. It was a week later and she still was not doing well. She would require surgery.

The difficulties created by her weight were aggravated because she was short. If you add enough weight into the surgical equation, it can turn it into a much more life-threatening event. People don't heal as well, it's harder to find a problem if there is one after surgery, and their pneumonias/blood clots/infections skyrocket. In addition, the sheer weight of their tissue tends to pull open the incision, even at the level of the muscle. Factor this all together and a routine operation can turn into a very big deal.

We took out the infected bowel, cleaned out the abscess, and completed the surgery. She did have wound issues after surgery. It would take us months to get the wound finally healed. Thankfully, the problems she had were above the level of the muscle and not life-threatening.

One early morning while waiting for a subsequent wound surgery, a figure appeared at the door of her room surrounded by bright light.

Then Anneka heard, "I'm looking for the dead woman."

She was having enough difficulties without seeing a bright light and having questions about "the dead woman."

"Wrong room!" Was all she could think to shout back. Later we would find out that one of the demented patients had gotten free and was roaming the halls. Needless to say, this well-placed rant had given Anneka quite a thrill.

We continue to work to diminish strange occurrences and problems in the hospital. Things are improving. When I operate on someone I know, I tell them that it seems like something unexpected always happens in the hospital. Fortunately, these events are usually minor nuisances. An imbalanced person making a weird comment would certainly fit that description.

> *If someone asks me if I'm the best, I always answer yes. I then tell them that I believe all surgeons think they are the best. Otherwise they couldn't do this job. I suggest they ask their regular doctor or someone else more neutral to give an opinion regarding me.*

# Lessons in Survival

Helen was going to have a big day. I didn't think she would survive.

The call came in about 9 PM on Saturday evening. I had been up the previous several nights and would eventually be up again a day or two later. The operating room staff was beginning to joke that 9 PM to 1 AM was my "block" time (assigned operating time).

The emergency room doctor said that her CT scan showed a bowel obstruction. My impression was that he added the fact that there was air in the intestine and the liver almost as an afterthought. I had to have him repeat it. This was an attention getter. We agreed that she needed emergency surgery and we started to make the preparations.

I drove in and looked at the CT scan myself. The gas in the tissue was dramatic, going along the stomach and up into the chest, and essentially filling the liver. It created so many artifacts/shadows in the scan that it actually made it hard to read.

It is generally taught that gas going into the vein toward the liver is a sign of terrible infection. Typically it's a gangrene type infection that creates this sort of gas. The general approach would be to separate the patient from the source of that infection. For example, if it were a bad appendix, you would need to get that appendix out in order for the patient to have a chance. If this principle held true, it would seem unlikely that the bad tissue could be removed from inside the chest, around the heart and lungs etc. It appeared to me to be a deadly combination.

And so I told this to Helen and to her family. She was about 80, thin, with a bloated and mildly tender stomach. Her blood pressure was dropping, her pulse very rapid at a hundred and eighty, and she was in acute renal failure. In spite of all this, she seemed mentally very clear and appropriate. So I told her and the family the findings. They noted that she had been to the doctor the day before. A scan had been ordered to be done in a few days from now. So it seemed she had gotten quite a bit sicker in the hours that had passed since then.

Essentially, I would do the best I could at surgery, but if my suspicions were true, it seemed less likely at best that she would survive. Everyone understood and agreed and Helen was prepared to go to surgery. A few quiet tears, and they let go of her hand so we could take her to the operating room.

Fortunately, my anesthesiologist didn't blink an eye. We each put in our own separate huge IVs, his at the neck and mine at the top of the leg. I told the operating room crew my suspicions. Nobody said much. We quickly prepared to operate.

With the abdomen open, it became apparent that there was a bowel obstruction. A thin loop of scar tissue had pinched the bowel closed. The bowel leading up to it was pretty enlarged but completely alive. The stomach had been stretched enormously, and the tube through the nose had drained out 6 to 7 liters of stomach juice. But the stomach was completely alive as well. In fact, other than a little mild edema (swelling in the tissue), everything seemed normal. Even the area where the bowel had been pinched was pink and "happy." Normally, a spot like that would at least have a bruise on it. When there's true gas in the tissue, it has a characteristic, crunchy feeling. The liver, stomach, and intestines all felt normal. Even though the liver looked normal, I did a small biopsy just to see if anything would show on the pathology report.

Interestingly enough, her pulse came down and her blood pressure went up with anesthesia. She almost immediately started to make urine. We were glad to see this, because typically anesthesia raises the heart rate and lowers the blood pressure. This is why starting a procedure on someone with poor vital signs can be daunting.

I was happy to report to the family that I did not find any gangrene. It was still hard to guarantee success, but at a minimum I now felt she had a chance, which had seemed less likely a few hours before based solely on my review of the CT scan. More quiet tears and a lot of gratitude for some good news.

Helen went on to recover fairly unremarkably. She had some unusual drainage about five days after surgery, so I repeated the CT scan. All the gas in the tissue and the liver was gone, and her CT scan looked normal for someone after surgery.

Just for effect, I pulled up the old scan for one of my radiologist friends.

"Oh, that lady died," he remarked.

Then I showed him the second CT scan. "She's doing quite well," I said. He looked back at the scans.

"Truth is stranger than fiction."

*****

I've heard of similar, but rare instances like this from other surgeons. In retrospect, something probably gets so distended that one of the layers ruptures and gas dissects in between the layers of the tissue. In this case it was probably the stomach. We occasionally see this in the fatty tissue of the body when we do laparoscopy in the abdomen. We blow up the abdomen with gas and insert a TV camera through tiny incisions to do the surgery in the abdomen. Occasionally, this gas will get out of the abdomen but not out of the skin. It will go through the layers of fatty tissue creating a very swollen look. Occasionally this will go through the whole body and all the way up to the face. The face can get very bloated looking with swollen eyelids and lips. If you push on it the tissue feels very crunchy. Once you stop the surgery, it all goes back to normal within an hour or two. I assume this is the same effect that happened on the inside of the abdomen for Helen.

So she gets to live another day. It's a reminder to me that so often in surgery I don't actually cure anything. I move things around to create an environment for healing, but it's really the marvelous body that does all the work. Even so, it's a tremendous privilege to be part of such a process.

> *One time in training, I had to tell the bride and family that the groom and best man died in a car wreck on the way to the wedding. I always try to pick the first words I tell them carefully, because I have a sense that those words will get "seared" into their memory. Opening words like "I have some bad news" or "We need to talk" helps them prepare to hear the heart-wrenching truth.*

# Stress Tolls

I was at home in my bedroom and I was hallucinating.

I woke up and looked over to see three people lying on carts. There were a lot of nurses working on the people on the first two carts. There was no one working on the man on the third cart. He was a larger man, lying face up, and naked.

I rolled over and woke up my wife. "The man on the third cart is dead," I told her. I rolled over and went back to sleep. She stared at me for a long time with wide eyes.

I was a second-year resident on the trauma service at our local County Hospital. We were on every other night call. I would leave for work at approximately 5 AM each day and return at approximately 5 to 6 PM the following evening, thirty six hours later.

My wife, Barb, was working the evening shift as a nurse. I would go to sleep until she came home around midnight, get up and have dinner with her, and sleep for a few more hours before I went back for my next 36 hour shift.

We had gotten married in March. I was nearing the end of a six-month run of every other night call. It was now August. In addition to hallucinating, there were other subtle tolls that the work would take on my life and my marriage, but somehow we survived these unusual circumstances.

Each of us residents would respond differently to the stress.

We found one of the women residents in a closet crying after she had been missing for two days.

Nearing the end of a difficult two-month stretch on neurosurgery with only two residents, one female colleague "couldn't take it anymore" and threw a very heavy old-fashioned cradle phone across the room, where it exploded. Tiny as she was, I didn't think she could have lifted it, let alone hurl it with such force.

The most dramatic example was probably the one that occurred during my rotation on the trauma service (the same service where I had been assigned at the time I had the hallucination).

It was the afternoon. The little nurses' station at the old County Hospital was around the corner from our tiny call room. The nurse came in and somewhat emphatically reminded another resident of a job he needed to finish. He sat for a moment without talking, then walked around the corner and shoved her. As I recall it, she shouted, "Call my lawyer, call the police!" and hit the floor.

The resident was fired. We went to the director expecting a replacement resident. True to County form at the time, they told us to fill in the gap ourselves. I finished the rotation on two out of three night call.

Needless to say, you cannot legally work those hours as a resident anymore. There are now laws that limit the hours. A typical law might require a limit of 80 hours a week and no more than 24 hours in a row.

When I was in training, you did "call" along with your other duties. *Call* meant you stayed in the hospital to be available for anything that could happen. (*Call*, after training when you have a job in General Surgery, means taking phone calls away from the hospital, while being available to go in to handle an emergency at any moment).

For instance, on transplant, we took *in house* (in the hospital) call every third night. We did our regular daytime duties and then handled all the nighttime problems every third night.

In addition to this call, transplant had its own unique requirement. The stickler was that if there was a liver transplant, the whole team stayed to provide extra staffing until it was done. Now, on third-night-call, you got one full 24 hours off every three weeks (when your day off landed on Sunday; Saturday morning was a required time in the hospital). But they would typically start a liver transplant on Friday night or Saturday morning.

These usually took about 36 hours at that time. We would take six hour shifts in the operating room to hold the abdomen open. This happened virtually every weekend. So we usually lost the one day off that we would have gotten every three weeks…

One of the second year residents told me of a fight he had once with this wife. She had complained that she wasn't getting enough love and attention from him. He answered that he was working on a different level with his scale of needs. She was operating at the higher level of love, but he was operating at the more basic level of food, sleep, and basic bodily functions. Needless to say, he quit surgery after his second year to go into something in medicine with more controlled hours (Radiation Oncology).

I interviewed at Duke during medical school for a position in surgery. The tradition there at the time was every-other-night call for the five years of in-hospital training, with several years of research in the middle of those years (in addition to the five years). One of the residents leading the tour was noted to say that a great resident was one who hated every-other-night call, because you would "miss half the good cases." Later in the day, someone (half jokingly) asked what the divorce rate was. "110 percent," was the answer, "because some people get married and divorced more than once during the training."

I have mixed feelings about the rigors of training in those days. I survived it, and I feel like I earned my own personal badge of honor. We were instilled with immense dedication and followed through on individual patient cases. In medicine today, it seems like the primary patient focus is slowly being diluted. The work is headed toward "shiftwork," with the patient becoming somebody else's problem when you go off shift. One might wonder if patient care will feel more fragmented to both patients and doctors in this new climate.

# Wooden Shoe Saves the Day

I was in surgery when I got the call.

I was at a hospital that I didn't go to very often. I did a surgery there once or twice a year on average at that time. I only went to that hospital if the patient's insurance required it or if it was a special request.

The emergency room paged me. The message was that they had a man, Stewart, with a swollen neck. The story wasn't entirely clear, but apparently he had recently had thyroid surgery. I was in the middle of a two to three hour surgery, so I was not emergently available.

I told the nurse to tell the emergency room to call the ER surgeon who was on call that day. Not only was I not available, but it was not my responsibility. The answer came back that the physician on call was not in the building and that they would wait for me. I strongly reiterated my request that they call the appropriate doctor, the one who was on call.

I didn't think much more about it. I assumed that they had "done the right thing."

As I was changing out of scrubs and into my street clothes, one of the orderlies in the operating room mentioned that they were still waiting for me downstairs in the emergency room. I assumed it had been taken care of, but was curious what was keeping that story going. It was at least an hour after they had first paged me and I'd not heard anything more about it. Certainly that problem would have been resolved by now...

Surgery was on the seventh floor. I took the elevator down to the ground floor, which would take me to my car. The emergency room was the last door on the left before I exited the building. I stuck my head in the door to make sure things were "under control."

I was greeted with the barrage that always sets me on edge. "We're so glad to see you. We've been waiting." (The other line that's hard for me to take is, "Are you in the building?" Because if I'm not in the building, I know that I will be shortly.) In any case, they had waited. It appeared that they had not called the other surgeon. I had that sinking feeling that something was unfolding and I was going to be involved whether I wanted to be or not.

I went around the corner to take a peek and see what was happening. Behind the curtain and taking up several of the emergency room stalls were approximately 15 people (various hospital employees), who mostly appeared to be standing and staring. The anesthesiologist had a scope in the patient's nose and was attempting to "get an airway." The patient was awake, sitting fairly upright with his head back. (When the airway is difficult, we purposely keep the patient awake until we can guarantee airway control.) He appeared to be thin overall, maybe a hundred and fifty pounds. And his neck was very swollen.

The crowd overall seemed mesmerized. I looked around and saw the charge nurse. I could see by the look in his eye that he understood the potentially dramatic nature of the moment. I whispered for a surgery tray, gloves, antiseptic, and a scalpel. He read my lips across the room and was back in seconds with equipment. He started setting up. The anesthesiologist was saying that basically he couldn't see anything in the back of the neck. The throat was too swollen on the inside.

When I had entered, I could hear the faintest breathing from the patient. Now, as the anesthesiologist quietly confirmed my suspicion that he could not get the breathing tube in, the patient took his last breath and passed out. The clock was running.

I sprayed the antiseptic on the neck, took the scalpel, and opened the recent incision. A whole lot of blood came out. The windpipe was now lying almost completely free in the middle of the incision. With the clock still running, I made an incision in the airway and slipped the breathing tube in. We immediately started giving oxygen by "bagging" the patient. The oxygen level we were monitoring in his blood came back and he woke up. We gave him some pain medication and put dressings on the neck. Then we called the operating room and told them that we would be up shortly to put things back together. I was then able to go home, as one of the surgeons from the original team came over and completed the surgery.

It turns out that the patient, Stewart was a close relative of one of the nurses at the hospital. She always called me "wooden shoe" because I was Dutch. He had just been discharged from an area hospital following thyroid surgery. They were in the car driving for about 10 miles when his neck swelled up and he was unable to breathe. They were in the vicinity of our hospital and that was how he ended up in the emergency room.

Stewart did well in the end. I was glad to hear the grateful response from the nurse, "Good work, wooden shoe."

Thinking back on this event reminds me never to assume that things are taking place according to one's own sense of logic, (especially where a hospital is concerned). This would be one of those days when the timing of events nudged me to remember that a "Grand Intelligence" was at work. In any case, I was thankful that on this particular day I was chosen to save the person who ended up under my care.

> *My senior partner once told me, "This job has a way of keeping you humble."*

# Attitude Adjustment

The patient was in the surgical intensive care unit. He was quite sick and waiting for a heart transplant.

At that time, it was the responsibility of the surgical resident (trainee) to draw all the blood work and do EKGs at any time other than the routine morning performances. So there we were, six of us trainees—two first-years, two second-years and two third-year residents—on this service trying to do our job. But the patient was cranky. When we would go into his room, he would yell at us. He would tell us were doing a terrible job. He would tell us what vein to use to draw blood and then yell at us if we didn't get it right. It wasn't unusual for the resident to be "thrown out of the room." We would be told to go right back in and get the job done.

One day, the patient developed a very fast heartbeat. It was picked up on the monitor outside of his room. As cardiac transplant patients, these people got a lot of attention. His room immediately filled up with people, preparing for resuscitation. The patient's heart rate was going approximately 180.

Someone at the front of the room called out, "We need to shock him. How much should we shock him with?"

Someone from the back of the room shouted "360."

The shock was given and the patient's heart rhythm returned to normal.

It turned out that the patient was wide awake when the shock was applied. The person at the front of the room knew this, but the person giving the dose from the back of the room did not know this. The shock level that was given was appropriate for an unconscious patient. The patient got the highest shock available.

Needless to say, the patient received a shocking experience in more ways than one.

From then on, however, the patient was as pleasant as could be.

"How can I help you? Is there anything I can do to make your job easier?"

Not the recommended way to get compliance, but as residents we were grateful for the change in attitude.

The experience reminded us of a story we had been told in a training session where we used electric shock paddles. The teacher made a point to remind us that the paddles we were using would be "live," with the power turned down as low as possible for our class. He mentioned that this was important to note because at one point one of the students had joked around and placed the paddles on his temples and pushed the button.

He knocked himself out.

Shock treatments are occasionally used in psychiatry for people with mental disorders. It's generally accepted that when these treatments work, the person becomes more "with it and happier." We wondered if it had had the same effect on the resident.

I'm not sure that the most dramatic example of attitude adjustment that I witnessed is legal. I was on the trauma training service at the time. With a significant trauma, the rule was that all clothes be removed and the patient underwent a brief but thorough examination. The current patient was angry and acting out, including spitting, kicking, biting, and hitting. Multiple people were doing their best to gain some control.

The resident running the area at the time did not care for trauma. He liked clean, orderly, daytime procedures that were scheduled in advance. Down and dirty on the front lines was not his style. I could see his blood pressure rising. He then walked over and took a syringe of muscle paralyzing medicine and pushed it into the IV. The patient quit moving.

I could hear the resident whisper in the patient's ear, "You'd better be calm when you wake up or I'll do this again."

He left the patient lying for a minute or two before they gave him some oxygen and re-stabilized him. The patient regained his ability to move a minute later. He was much calmer, if not entirely helpful. We could get on with our work of taking care of him.

Protecting the staff and protecting the patient simultaneously in these situations can be a dilemma. I was glad for the assistance the chief resident gave us, but was a little uncomfortable with his methods. Needless to say, I never saw the technique used again. We were thankful, however, for the subsequent cooperation we received from the patient. We were able to do our job that day knowing no one would be unnecessarily bruised or bitten.

> *One of my surgeon friends had a patient tell him, as he was preparing to go to sleep on the operating room table, "If something goes wrong, I'll sue you." The doctor took him off the table, told him to find a new surgeon, and sent him home.*

# Guatemala Adventure

Guatemala "missionary" surgery trips began with a one-hour plane trip from Guatemala City. We never knew if it would be cloudy at the pass in the mountains until we got there. The adventure was that if it was cloudy, the plane would have to turn around and take us back where we started. We would then need to take a 12 hour bumpy bus ride to the same destination.

I would eventually make four one-week Guatemala trips. Luckily, I never had to take the bus.

The natives were kind and deeply grateful for the work we did. They would sometimes walk days for the chance to have us do their surgery.

We would set up shop in an old semi-deserted hospital apparently built by the Americans. The structure was good, but almost everything had been stolen out of it. The water tower was still standing, but we would have to get it running again when we got there.

The only thing that was ever stolen from us was two bottles of mint jelly. We planned to use this for our final big dinner before we left.

We would routinely have all the patients sign a consent form. I once asked the director of the missionary program what they did with the paperwork. "We throw it out at the end of the week," came the reply. So much for protocol.

We didn't have any facility or equipment to do lab work. After discussing the patient's health (via three different interpreters), we would look in their eye lid to determine if their blood count was okay. A pink inner eyelid was a good sign.

The operating was fairly primitive. One of the rooms where we worked was actually an old bathroom. There was only room enough for the surgeon and one assistant. The anesthesiologists would administer the spinal anesthesia and then leave. In the afternoon when the electricity was weak (the "brownout"), the assistant would also have to hold a flashlight. I have a vivid memory of opening the belly and performing a tubal ligation under such circumstances.

One young man felt he had a lump in his abdomen. Sure enough, when he lay down I thought I could feel it. We discussed it as fully as possible, and he understood that we would make an incision in his abdomen and attempt to remove it.

There was always some trepidation on our part in these cases. If there were permanent injury or (heaven forbid!) death from one of our surgeries, it would have negative consequences for the program and the possibility of future visits. Still, we believed we should try to help this young man, and we prepared him for surgery.

Once he was asleep, I made the incision. No mass. Nothing. I was feeling around more and more. Meanwhile, the anesthesiologist, who had as much invested in this case now as I did, started to raise an eyebrow from the other side of the surgical drape.

"What's happening? TFS ('trapped fart syndrome')? Did you really feel something? What's going on?"

And then I found it, pushed off to the side, about the size of my fist. The mass was attached to the blood vessels for the intestine, enabling it to move around dramatically. I was able to take it out without any further difficulty. It appeared to be a mass from a river fluke.

He went on to recover uneventfully. I went on to recover uneventfully.

At another time, I was doing a minor surgery for an ingrown toenail. As (bad!) luck would have it, the scalpel went through his toenail and into my thumb. It gave me a cut about 1/2 inch long, near the base of my thumbnail. There was copious blood flowing and that part of my thumb went numb, so unfortunately I had cut both my artery and nerve.

On this particular trip I was with one other surgeon, a urologist. I asked him to stitch me up, and for whatever reason, he declined. I got the feeling he probably had never stitched up a laceration before. I held pressure for a while, then kept a tight Band-Aid on the wound. Even though there was some fat sticking out, it healed beautifully, just like any other cut I've seen. After that experience, I understood that maybe stitches aren't always as necessary as I thought for healing to take place.

I hoped there wasn't going to be any hepatitis or other blood issues that would arise regarding my cut. We had no way to test the patient and I couldn't get any testing done until I got home (by that time I'd forgotten about it). It's now years later, and everything seems to have turned out okay....

The experience created a sort of badge of honor for me. Now, any time a patient experiences a "minor" nerve issue after surgery (an area of numbness due a clipped nerve), I point to my scar and the area of numbness to reassure them that it won't be a problem..

We would essentially have only the supplies we brought with us on those trips. One year we forgot to take masks. At first we made them out of hats or shoe covers, but by the end of the week we literally gave up on using them at all. Sometimes when I look back on these circumstances, I wonder if all our fussing and rules for surgery may not be as important as we're led to believe.

People sometimes ask me about the reputation of the facility where I work, or another facility they may be considering for their surgery. They want to make sure the conditions will be supportive for the procedure they need to have done. As I think back on those Guatemala days, I tell people to pick their surgeon carefully. If he is comfortable with his working conditions, everything else can reasonably be expected to fall into place.

# A Day at the Office

The schedule was going to take a beating at the office this day.

Olivia was 26 and had found the breast cancer herself. On the office schedule we have allowed 15 minutes.

"Better warn people I may be a little late."

It was a larger lump. She had her x-rays and biopsy. We went through her options: chemotherapy first, lumpectomy, breast removal. Reconstruction may or may not be necessary. She would need other x-rays to look for cancer spread. Gene cancer testing. Chemotherapy could take away her chance for children in the future. Possible ovary egg harvest beforehand. "Portacath" may take surgery as well. There was no hurrying this conversation. We finished up. Some crying. Some handholding.

On to the next room, Isabel. Yeah. A breast biopsy postop check. This should be quick. 45 years old and benign findings on recent biopsy. The incision looks good. Time to go.

She asks "My previous biopsy had atypia. Do I need more surgery?"

Still not difficult. "No you could start with a risk evaluation" (enough risk and you could consider mastectomy or other treatments).

"My mammogram is hard to read and I worry about it. My mother had breast cancer and it stays on my mind. She died from the cancer." I couldn't postpone her needed discussion about mastectomy, reconstruction, and all the possible options and implications. Another hour behind.

Trudy. A breast abscess returning for her visit after surgery.

My work is quite varied, but today would be breast day. At least an abscess should be quick. The site of the abscess was healing okay, but the other side was starting to get red. She had a lot of pain on and off for months in various areas of her breast. She had already had multiple procedures. Her last pathology showed *periductal mastitis*. An unclear process, the body probably turns on itself and creates inflammation. It can be very difficult to treat. In principle, we work very hard to avoid big surgeries like mastectomy (breast removal). She wanted to know all about it. She wanted to know what we would do if the inflammation would not go away. She wanted to know about mastectomy and reconstruction. On top of that, I had been sued for offering mastectomy in a radical case with similar issues. A little sweating on my part. We worked through it. Another hour behind.

*****

In general, my patients are saints. There was no complaining to me that day. The receptionist did extra work to keep people informed, but overall they were accepting of the delay. Most of them were still quite pleasant. I apologized to each new patient. Occasionally I offered, "Be thankful you're not the reason I'm late."

It's amazing to me what patients go through from another standpoint as well. They come to see me with a life-changing issue like breast cancer and immediately we have to address surgery or surgeries, chemotherapy, radiation therapy, all the testing, options for reconstruction and so forth. The focus is on getting through all the aspects of treatment, any one of which would be daunting. Underneath it all is the fact that they are also needing to come to terms mentally and emotionally with their diagnosis, but the frenzy of treatment often delays this from happening. I occasionally see patients later in their course of treatment, often during radiation. At this point, the worst is over and they are on the road to recovery, yet they tell me they feel exhausted. I gently offer that I wonder if, after all the surgery and decisions related to their recovery, they are finally dealing with the underlying issues and the mental exhaustion of adapting to this new phase in their life.

# Blood and Blindness

It was a long night on the transplant service.

I was busy through the entire night. Patients were critically ill. I was a second-year surgery resident at the time. Mostly kidney and liver transplant patients, they were often the sickest of the sick.

I was barely keeping up this particular evening. The nurse mentioned more than once that one of the patients, John J., had blood in his urine. He had undergone a kidney transplant. As I triaged my way through the night, he stayed lower on my list. As long as the blood in the urine kept moving, it was rarely a sign of significant complications. If the amount of blood in the urine was significant, it would clot, but then it would stop moving and cause more pain. Other than that, it was rare for someone to have their blood count drop much just from blood in the urine.

Some time during the night I told the nurse to draw a blood count, set some blood aside, and keep me posted.

So I finally entered John J.'s room just as my team arrived to start the new day. His room was the first room we entered as we started rounds.

Just as we entered the room, he said, "I can't see."

At about the same moment, the nurse came in and said hemoglobin is 1.6. Just to be clear, a normal hemoglobin is 12 to 14. When I was in training we would give blood for a count that got as low as 8 to 10. We still generally give blood when the count is below seven.

It wasn't entirely clear how his blood count got that low, but low it was. And the patient was clearly symptomatic (blind!).

My chief resident was a man of direct action. The nurse mentioned that the blood was ready, but that the paperwork was not. The chief ran through the hospital and down the long stairwell directly to the blood bank. Somehow he managed to meet the blood bank personnel with the blood but without the paperwork. He grabbed the blood, leaving the blood bank person a little dismayed, and ran back to the room. He started the blood himself and squeezed it in by hand.

As he finished squeezing in the second pint, the patient said "I can see again."

I'd never heard of anything like that happening before, and I've never seen anything like it since. This would be the lowest blood count survivor of my career. A potentially grim outcome was averted, and I was happy that John J. survived.

The other residents gave me some interesting looks that morning. I don't think I bothered to try to defend it. It had been one heck of a night.

\*\*\*\*\*

What that experience did buy me was a distinguished spot on the "wall of shame."

There was a large bulletin board in the resident "on call" room. On it were listed an informal collection of the different incidents that had happened over the years on the transplant service. In a sense, I suppose this sounds disrespectful. As I look back on it, however, I have come to view it as just the opposite. In my mind it's become a "wall of fame."

Transplant service is a tribute to the fight for life. These people are sicker and more willing to risk everything to buy some time than a lot of other people in the hospital. With all that they go through, including thin blood that doesn't clot easily, immuno-suppression, troubles with infections, and various surgeries, they are a setup for problems.

Just as an example, we would often have to place big IVs into large veins on people whose blood had no clotting capability. Fortunately, this usually went well. These people needed this assistance. Occasionally, however, in spite of our best efforts, people had bleeding. One of my colleagues earned his place on the wall of shame when the patient required 6 pints of blood after his IV placement. Of course, he had done the best he could under the circumstances.

So I got my spot on the wall of shame. To my recollection, it's the only time I've heard of someone losing their sight as a result of low blood count. I think I was as relieved as John J. was when his sight returned.

> *I occasionally ride my motorcycle without a helmet and get chided by my medical colleagues. One day in the operating room, I got stuck with a needle from an AIDS patient. I was supposed to take anti-AIDS medicine for a month, but I could only tolerate it for a week (it exhausted me). It occurrs to me that I face far more risk at work (HIV, hepatitis, losing a lawsuit and having my savings taken away, etc) than I do when riding my motorcycle.*

# Eat a Big Breakfast

I was facing a big surgery. I had been preparing a man, Andreas, with a chronic problem for his surgery. The planned surgery would be lengthy. He was now in the hospital with a bleeding ulcer. He was unstable and needed surgery for this new issue as well.

I was a relatively new "attending surgeon" sitting with my senior partner eating breakfast. I had been stabilizing the patient through the night. My partner and I never needed to talk much. In fact, from the day we began working together, we rarely discussed anything. When we covered for one another, he would always do what I would have wanted, and I assumed I always did what he would have expected. It seemed often times that we didn't even say hello in the morning. I think we both really liked it this way.

So I was eating breakfast with him, contemplating my surgical challenge. I described the underlying issue. The patient would need his intestines rearranged and a bypass to the bile duct. This could be a delicate procedure that would often take more than a few hours. But his bleeding ulcer demanded that I remove a third of his stomach, also requiring a reroute of the intestines. I hoped there might be some magic.

I ran the litany of issues past my senior partner, and waited for his words of wisdom.

He contemplated, then offered "Eat a big breakfast."

I considered that for a few minutes, then let it go. It turned out to be good advice. The ulcer surgery went well and I was able to complete both procedures. However, it took me about eight hours, so I needed the big breakfast.

Andreas did okay after surgery. I had concern about a leak at the bile duct hook up, and left his drain in as a backup safety guard. The patient was tall and soft-spoken. His career was going from bar to bar picking up empty beer cans and selling them. He went home with his drain in, and I often imagined him on his rounds with the drain taped to the side.

I left that drain in long enough that it wore a hole in the colon. A frustrating problem, it's called an *enterocutaneous fistula*. After such a "fancy job," this was a bit of a hard pill to swallow. I reviewed the new problem with him. As usual, he didn't say very much and seemed pretty accepting. The good news was that the drain had been there so long it created its own track. I was able to take the drain out and that track closed. I thought I had won.

Andreas then came back in with diarrhea. He had lost a little weight. Pretty nonspecific. In any case, we worked him up. He now had an opening from the beginning of the intestine to the colon. My drain had apparently worn into two pieces of bowel and there was now an opening between them. This one required surgery. I took him back and fixed the fistula.

It always amazes me where the winding road surgery can take me and the patient. I imagine Andreas out collecting beer cans, hopefully no worse for the wear. When I have a rather daunting case, however, the advice of my partner still rings true to me, "Eat a big breakfast."

> *When I first joined my senior partner, he said, "We'll split call evenly. I took the first 30 years!" (He was joking, of course. We did split the call evenly: we each took every other night.)*

# Karma

Something new.

It was Saturday afternoon in Guatemala where we were doing missionary surgery. The woman who came to see us had stool draining in her groin. On examination she had a perfectly formed *ileostomy* (bowel draining to the surface of the skin).

I had just finished residency/training and was taking the opportunity "before children" for a travel/missionary trip/adventure "vacation." We were just beginning to unpack our things when this woman, Flora, showed up at the door. A Guatemala native, she used her beautiful multicolored hand woven cloth to catch the stool. It took three interpreters each way to translate through the multiple dialects. Eventually it became clear that she had experienced an incarcerated groin hernia. It had died and sloughed, leaving her with the ileostomy. An incarcerated (stuck) hernia left untreated would generally be expected to be lethal! So this was unusual and pretty amazing.

It would take one week to do the surgery and get her through recovery. Typically, intestinal recovery after bowel surgery took five to seven days. If we waited until Monday, she would likely not recover by the time we left. So we decided to set up and do the surgery that night. We opened the belly and put the two ends of the bowel back together.

Our "recovery room" was close quarters. Each patient got only a small place to rest. The family would stay with the patient and help with the recovery. There were multiple little huddles all over as patients regained strength enough to be able to leave. Eventually the story of Flora's intestinal surgery got around and everyone began to wait for a bowel movement. When this great event came, the whole recovery room full of patients and families cheered and celebrated for this woman who had not had a normal bowel movement in a long time.

At approximately the same time as Flora's recovery, a man in his early 30s fell off a cliff gathering sticks. He broke his back and was paralyzed. His family included several small children. We felt terrible and offered plans to take him back to Guatemala City. Both he and his wife declined. They had no money. They had no resources. She would not be able to visit him there. It would not be possible for him to be useful again in his old life. In the end they declined all therapy. We left him on a bed in another part of the recovery room. She took care of him. He declined food and was dying as we left. They worked it out. She would remarry as soon as possible to continue on with her life.

It was a stark example to me that some get to live and some get to die, some we can help, and some we cannot.

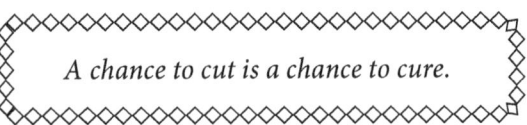

*A chance to cut is a chance to cure.*

# Bad Day

It was a Labor Day holiday. A patient of my partner and mine, Ted, had had multiple surgeries and now was back in the hospital. He had been admitted several days ago, critically ill. He had since gotten a little better. After checking him over and considering the data from all the tests that had been done, it looked to me to be a bad gallbladder.

The next day all the regular doctors came back after the holiday. I received several phone calls from them. On their review, they didn't feel it was his gallbladder (I still thought it was). I was told he didn't need any surgery. Not really bothersome, and yet I could feel a little twinge inside me. Not only was I indirectly being told I was wrong, but I remained concerned about the patient. I just hoped it would get figured out correctly.

The next phone calls I remember were regarding a mildly complicated patient of mine, Stacey. I had removed her gallbladder and left a drainage tube in her bile duct. She continued to have some lingering pain from pancreatitis that had been set off by her gallstones. With my drainage tube in place, it was clear that her problem had been taken care of. Within an hour, however, two different doctors called me with concerns that the drainage tube was inadequate. They thought she needed another procedure. From a surgeon's standpoint, it was pretty straightforward. She had the correct drainage for her to be able to heal and I didn't believe she needed an additional procedure by the gastroenterologist. I felt a little annoyed at being "corrected."

Later in the same day, I was in the office. I had a late middle-aged gentleman, Andrew, who needed his dialysis access moved to his arm. (The first place you put the access us a catheter in the shoulder. This typically goes bad after a couple of years.) He was quite concerned, and appeared to actually be afraid of it because he had heard from other patients that complications can occur with the access in the arm. I spent a long time with him going over and over the concepts until he became comfortable with the idea of placing the access in his arm. I was glad to be able to help, but it left me quite late to see my other cases in the office.

As I came out of the room, I heard the woman in the second exam room say, "Is he always this late? It's been an hour. I've never seen someone so late. Does he operate as poorly as he manages his time? I have to go to the bathroom. I better not be out of the queue when I come back. I can't believe this!"

My happiness over helping the previous gentleman melted away. She came back, and I apologized for the delay. We were able to move on and she was happy with the answers I gave her regarding her hernia.

All in all, there was nothing dramatic; it was just one of those not so great days.

My office building at that time was adjacent to the hospital, so at the end of the day I was in the physician's locker room completing a few things when the open-heart surgeon came around the corner. He was a little younger, normally pleasant and happy, very conscientious, and very talented.

"How was your day?" I asked.

"Not so hot," he answered, with the slightest hint of "glum." That was out of character for him, and I raised an eyebrow.

He went on to say, "My first patient coded (heart stopped) as we put her to sleep this morning. She had a known valve problem. (Occasionally these kinds of problems happen in that scenario.) We had to do heart massage. First we did it with her intact, then I opened the chest and did more heart massage. She's alive, but she's not waking up so far."

My compassion went out to him. What could I say? We've all been in that scenario. It's a long walk down the hall to talk to the family.

I thought back on my day. There is a bad day. And then there's a *bad day*. The nuisance level of problems like doctor politics, my ego, and patient issues didn't seem to be quite as big a deal after being reminded of the life-and-death issues that we deal with as surgeons.

---

*It is very hard for me to be friendly after a patient dies unexpectedly, or something similar happens. People are friendly where I work and a lot of them know me. It takes a lot of effort for me to return a happy greeting when I feel miserable, frustrated, and sad inside. The same applies when I walk into my house on one of those days. For people who can understand, I try to give them a heads-up that I "need a little space."*

# Jake the Motorcycle Man

I felt like I recognized this man.

I was a second year resident assigned on the trauma unit at County as he was rolled in with a broken leg.

Our schedule on the trauma unit was to take front room call every four nights and back room call every four nights. These calls alternated so that we would be there every other night.

It turned out I had first admitted him four nights ago after a motorcycle accident. We had placed him in the recovery ward on the third floor.

Apparently he decided to leave by jumping out the third floor window. He broke his leg.

The ambulances at the county hospital at the time would drive into the drop off area in the back of the building. When the drop off was complete, they could drive on through, exiting in the same direction.

As the ambulance left the drop off area, they found my "motorcycle man" on the ground below his window. They "scooped" him up, drove around the block, and pulled back into the drop off area.

So there he was, being rolled in once again into the trauma unit. I was a little confused, feeling like I recognized him. It took me a few minutes to get the story and figure things out.

"Nice to see you again," I said to Jake.

# Life on Call

The call for the appendectomy came at 1:00 in the afternoon.

Not a big deal. The case technically didn't even fall to me. But I was still in the building. Easily done. It was Thanksgiving Day and I called the team in.

The next call came at 6:00 PM for a rectal abscess and I was now at home. This patient, however, had drunk CT dye, which technically gave me an excuse to delay the surgery. Normally, we would drain an abscess immediately when it was found. But generally we try to avoid anesthesia if someone's put something in their stomach in the last six hours. So I gave the order to get the patient a room. I would see him in the morning and take care of it then.

The next call came for a feeding tube that was out. The emergency room doctor had partially put it back in. On x-ray it may or may not be in the correct position. It's a nice thing to fix sooner rather than later, but it could wait until morning. "Just tape it down" and I would check on it later.

The next call of consequence came at midnight. It was a woman, Frances, whose CT scan said that she had blood in her belly.

"What's the blood count?"

"17" came the answer from the emergency room. This was actually higher than normal, and not consistent with bleeding.

"How long ago did you check this hemoglobin?"

"Seven hours ago."

"How are the vitals?"

"Stable. No problem."

All in all, these findings didn't seem to add up. A possible CT showing bleeding, but no other signs. There was also a question of bladder thickening on the CT.

Midnight.

The inevitable surgeon's question. "Do I get out of bed?"

If there really was blood in the belly (which seemed questionable to me), the most definitive reason for surgery would be the bleeding, along with a patient's vital sign instability. But there was no instability now. It seemed reasonable to repeat the blood count and send her to the ICU, so I followed this course of action and didn't get out of bed. Staying in bed is nice, but I usually find my sleep isn't very sound under these circumstances…

When it was finally sorted out, Frances never required any surgery. It took us a couple days to confirm this. In the end, she had no blood in the belly. It was a swollen, irritated bladder that we treated with IV antibiotics.

\*\*\*\*\*

Sometimes the ER doc can make it pretty painless.

"It's an appendix. You should do it now."

Other times it's not quite so simple. This can be especially true for someone newer at the job.

"I have a patient. The history includes diabetes and hypertension."

It would be the middle of the night now, and I start to groggily think, *Hmm… maybe a diabetic foot. Won't have to get out of bed.*

"They have right lower quadrant pain."

*Oh-oh. Appendicitis. I'll have to get out of bed.*

"We ordered the CT. While we waited, the pain moved to the right upper quadrant."

*Yeah. Gallbladder. Tomorrow. I get to sleep.*

"The white blood count is 24,000."

*Oh-oh. That sounds more serious. Maybe it will have to be done now.*

"The CT scan shows (*here it comes*) uncomplicated

diverticulitis." *I get to sleep.*

Except now I'm so jazzed I can't fall back to sleep for a couple of hours.

People ask me, "How's your call?" When the call is okay, I answer that it's good. The problem is I never know if it was a good call until it's over.

Call reminds me of the story of "so far so good." The guy jumps out of the window of a 100 story building and as he goes by each floor, people hear him say "so far so good." So that is often my answer now to people who ask how my call is going: "So far so good."

Call makes me irritable. I don't go out much anymore while on call. Not only do I dislike being called away from the scheduled activity, but I'm generally snarky enough that I'm just no fun. I think my wife and kids have learned to recognize the pattern. I generally lie pretty low when on call to avoid creating more aggravation for myself or others.

*****

In the end, call is about helping somebody who's hurting. This may be no more true in any field than general surgery. In general surgery there is quite often an acute problem that involves pain. I continue to find gratification in helping someone in this situation correct the problem and get back to their life.

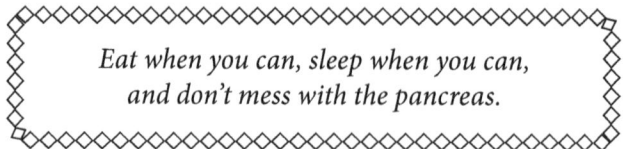

*Eat when you can, sleep when you can, and don't mess with the pancreas.*

# Fun Yet?

I was the attending (responsible) surgeon at the time and the resident assigned to me for teaching was not impressed with me.

When I would give a suggestion or an order for a patient, I noted some unexpressed and expressed skepticism from the resident. It didn't bother me a lot. But it did register that, at a minimum, this resident didn't have much respect for my abilities or approach.

At various times in my career, I've had residents working with me. Overall, I love teaching. It's not conveying the book learning that intrigues me so much. It's the experiences and the human part of surgery that I love to share. It's teaching how to handle the patient's issue as well as the patient's personality and perspective.

A woman, Holly, came into the emergency room with known metastatic cancer. She was in a life threatening situation of bleeding into her belly. The scan revealed a single tumor in the left side of the liver and it appeared that this was the source of the bleeding in the abdomen. The size of this piece of cancer that had come back was approximately the size of a volleyball. By size alone, the problem could be daunting. However, in its location on the left lobe of the liver, it was possible it would be easy to get to.

If the area of bleeding turned out to be accessible, we would solve the bleeding problem by placing a few stitches in the area. Then the patient would be stabilized and placed in the ICU to determine the next course of action to treat her tumor. If the source of the bleeding was not accessible to simple suturing, we would remove that entire section of the liver containing the tumor. Relative to the size of the liver, the area of attachment to the liver was not very big. If a resection were required, there would be a short time when it would get more bloody. But overall, such a case shouldn't be particularly difficult.

We stabilized her and went up to surgery. The resident would assist me as I navigated a way to get control of the bleeding. We quietly began our work. I didn't linger on talking about the approach we would use.

At the time, I didn't give much thought to the effect such a case might have on my relationship with a resident. In general, my approach is just to do my work in a case like this and have the person helping me observe. This kind of teaching by demonstration doesn't require a lot of talking. The case would speak for itself.

We made the incision and opened the abdomen. There was quite a lot of blood. It was at about this point the resident started to get very quiet. I cleaned it out per routine. The tumor was bleeding from the inside and oozing out to the surface, so the only option was to remove it. I placed a few preliminary stitches, and then cut the tumor off from the edge of the liver.

Immediately there was again a lot of bleeding. I controlled it with my hand.

I've developed a habit over the years when things are a bit dramatic but not out of control. I looked up and asked the resident, like I've done before in similar situations, "Are we having fun yet?"

He now looked pale as a ghost and wasn't talking. I went on to apply the final stitches to control the bleeding. The patient did fine.

From then on, that resident treated me like I was some sort of a god. It was as if I could do no wrong and he savored everything that I tried to teach. I enjoyed working with him so much more after that case.

*****

When things get intense in the OR, I tend to get more quiet.

I'm sure this is a little frustrating for the staff, because eventually I get so quiet that it's hard for them to hear me. They never complain, and when I get the wrong instrument handed me, I just know to speak up a little more.

Over time, the nurses learn to read me. If I'm in a bigger case with a veteran nurse and say "better call for some blood," I'll see him or her start scrambling. They drop everything, get the blood, get help, "mobilize for war."

If it's not a veteran nurse, she won't understand the subtlety of this request or the significance of the fact that it is generally a warning that things could get rough. A lot of times they'll linger or be distracted. The addition of a little more information, telling them to get help and get moving, is usually sufficient for them to understand that the call for blood is often a prelude to more intensity.

A ruptured spleen is another case that also offers a sense of drama. Fortunately, the spleen is attached on a stalk that is tucked away, but in most cases it is easy to get to. It gives that same sense of excitement, but if you know how to bring it up and grab the blood vessels, it's reasonably easily controlled. If the liver case had not come up with my resident, it's likely a ruptured spleen would have done the job just as well.

> *Surgery takes a strange combination of ego and restraint. You must believe you are the best at surgery, but make sure that you don't carry this attitude over into everything else in your life.*

# Midnight Bleeder

I was a little aggravated.

The phone call came around midnight. I could hear quite a bit of commotion at the other end. People were speaking loudly, and there were quite a few of them. It was hard to understand my caller. In the background I could hear "Try to stop the bleeding!" and "Get the emergency cart!" My wife was already awake, but I decided to leave the room so I could speak loudly enough to be heard.

Let me preface my remarks by saying that I don't like getting out of bed at night. Probably most people feel this way. But I'll admit that some of my colleagues seem to handle it without much fanfare. In any case, it's hard for me to be up for hours in the middle of the night and function the next day. It's not the surgery necessarily, it's having enough energy to be adequately kind to myself, the staff, and the patients. When I start to get short, it's fairly noticeable. In addition, I get headaches fairly easily. A short night of sleep or no sleep can often set one off. On top of all that, if the bad night comes early in the week, I sometimes feel I don't recover until a day or two after I finally get a break. It can make for a long week, especially on a week that has late evenings already built-in.

Eventually I was able to discern from the caller that it was a dialysis patient with a bleeding access. This "access" can either be the vein previously connected to an artery or a plastic tube between artery and vein. These are typically in the arm. The blood in these conduits is essentially under arterial pressure. To perform dialysis, they place two large needles through the skin into this vein or plastic tube (the plastic tube is buried completely under the skin) and dialyze the patient for several hours. Afterwards, they remove the needles and put pressure on the area. Occasionally the needle site can bleed and this can be aggravated if the access is starting to develop blockages. It is not unusual to get a call related to "prolonged bleeding" when the access starts to deteriorate.

As an emergency "surgery," in most cases this situation is not particularly difficult to get under control. The key is to understand that there is a "tube" underneath the skin that is bleeding. In a calm setting, you can even walk a novice through this repair.

But now I was yelling on the phone, "Can you hear me?"

"Don't slip on the blood! Get a blood pressure cuff!"

I tried again. "Get out of the room so you can hear me."

"What? What?"

"Put your finger on the tube near the bleeder! Then it will slow down so you can put a stitch in it," I tried to offer.

"I can't hear you." I quickly tried several more times to help them understand. It wasn't clear that I was making any progress.

It's easier to get out of bed when it's a problem that really requires a surgeon. To know there is someone standing next to the patient who could most likely handle the problem added to my aggravation. I'd had a long week, and it was a little tougher than usual for me to sort out my personal feelings from my job requirement to meet the needs of this situation. In any case, we were making no progress. They needed me. I quickly got dressed and started my drive to the hospital.

A short distance away from my destination, I got a page. Answering the phone, a very calm, collected nurse told me that the stitch was in and everything was okay. I was now at the entrance to the hospital. I pulled over to the side of the road and rested my head back against the head rest. I went from sleeping to partially terrorized and yelling to the "long" (ten minute) drive in my car with my heart pounding to "by the way, everything's fine – we don't need you anymore."

*Michael DeHaan*

I try to avoid making changes in my approach to work based on a single bad event. In surgery these come and go with relative frequency. They're almost never reproducible, although the heart pounding I experience seems fairly constant. However, as I sat there contemplating my twenty minutes of chaos, I decided something had to give. About a day later, I decided to drop my third day of office hours. This would allow me a little time midweek for recovery from these unanticipated but surprisingly frequent projections into my life. It gave me a quiet comfort to do something positive to regain a little sanity.

> *People sometimes complain to me about another doctor. I tell them to get a new doctor. Doctors come in all different abilities and personalities. Life is short. Don't struggle with a doctor you don't get along with.*

## Two Whipples

The Whipple procedure is a big surgery. We take out part of the stomach and intestine, part of the pancreas, part of the bile duct, and hook everything back together. The Whipple can be done for various reasons, but it is most commonly performed to remove a tumor/cancer in this area near the top of the abdomen. I had one scheduled on a Friday. As the schedule turned out, it would be followed by another surgery to go into the abdomen and look for recurrent cancer.

There was an amazing story that I was able to verify over the years. My senior partner had done two "Whipples" in the same morning before lunch. I was not as quick, and my surgeries typically took six to eight hours each.

I was finished with the first surgery on Elena in the mid-afternoon. I received a call to look at a hernia in the ER. I went down and made the necessary plans. No surgery was required that day for this hernia.

I then undertook the second procedure, to investigate for possible recurrent cancer in a patient, Fernando. As the surgery progressed, I realized that this patient would need a "Whipple" procedure as well. There was recurrent cancer, but it was localized only to the first part of the intestine. We finished up the surgery and I went home.

So, I accomplished my two Whipples in one day and got home about 3 AM.

I was tired. As my head touched the pillow, the phone rang.

"Was I coming to see the hernia in the ER?"

"I already did," I answered, perhaps more curtly than I would have liked. I explained I had seen the patient at 3 PM and had taken care of the issue.

They said, "No, there was a second hernia waiting for the past six hours. Hadn't I gotten the message?" I could hardly believe my ears and made them repeat it. Yes, I would need to go back in.

I got dressed and went back to the ER. I asked the patient how long he had been hurting and he told me it had been approximately six months. This was not much of an emergency. The patient had waited six hours for me to see him, and I'd gotten out of bed exhausted to inform him that his surgery could wait. Our discussion about this didn't take long. I gave him my number so he could call the office and schedule the surgery. Needless to say, I don't think I ever saw him again.

So many things can happen in medicine so fast that it's amazing there isn't more confusion. Fortunately, this day ended with only a bit of sore feelings and not much more. I was glad to get back home and finally rest.

> *People say to me, "I don't like _____ (fill in the blank: needles, proctoscopy, surgery).*
> *I tell them, "The people who worry me are the people who* like *(needles, proctoscopy, surgery)."*

## Symptoms and Outcomes

Things don't always end up where you expect.

Alicia originally came in with swollen legs. An eventual CT scan showed a tumor in her abdomen that appeared to extend backwards around the big blood vessel that drains the blood from her legs. At first glance this would appear to be hopeless.

She was about 40. She was the front office person for our local police department. In spite of her problems, she smiled as I described some of my encounters with the officers that she worked with. At one point, a friend of mine was helping us move to a new house a block away from our current home. We were driving a loaded pickup truck through the alleys when we were surrounded by four or five cop cars and police starting to pull out their guns. One of them said we were trying to outrun them (he had called for backup). Even the other officers had to smile when this claim was made. I don't think our loaded truck ever went over 5 miles per hour! It reminded me of Barney Fife, the bumbling deputy of Mayberry from the Andy Griffith show.

In any case, we got them to reopen the blood vessel to her legs in radiology. Next, I took her to surgery. Thankfully, the original tumor was not very large and I cut out the piece of small bowel that was involved. It was still frustrating in surgery that I couldn't do more to help remove the apparent extension of tumor to the back of the abdomen.

It turned out, however, that the majority of the reaction in the back of the abdomen was a scar type response set off by the tumor. With removal of the original tumor, she actually had some shrinkage of this scar type response. In the end, her cancer would be quite sensitive to chemotherapy. In spite of tumor in the liver and the extensive tumor response in the back of her abdomen, she would go on to live a normal life for a long time after that.

I would not have guessed that swollen legs would lead to an intestinal tumor. And when I saw the scan, I wouldn't have guessed that she could have a normal life again for even a short period of time, let alone for many years.

*****

Another woman, Elearnor, came to see me for hernia. She was elderly and the mother of one of my good friends who is a nurse. She said she'd been having increased pain down by her groin. She pointed toward her abdomen and said she had a hernia.

In the examination, her stomach seemed stretched out to me, but I couldn't find a hernia. She wasn't overweight, so I didn't think I was missing anything. It is always disconcerting to me when a patient says they have something and I can't find it. I offered her a CT scan, and we made the arrangements.

The scan showed a mass in the bones of her back and a small lesion in the kidney. In the final analysis, she had a cancer that had gone from the kidney to her vertebrae. I was correct, no hernia. With the outcome that unfolded, I wish it had been a hernia for her. I never would have guessed that a suspicion about a groin hernia would end up leading to and revealing a spreading kidney tumor.

*****

My most memorable "no hernia there" story took place during a morning clinic. My wife Barb was working with me at the time as my office nurse. It was not unusual for me to get behind schedule during clinic mornings, and most people were tolerant about this. One fellow, however, was becoming notably impatient as the morning progressed. Eventually I shuffled the schedule around and had Tony brought back to the exam room. Barb reported that he seemed extremely agitated, so I went in to see what was going on.

Tony told me he had a hernia and that he needed to have it repaired quite soon. I took a look at him and noted that he was quite thin. He was standing and a true hernia would have been obvious. I couldn't see a hernia. I carefully asked him where it was and he vaguely pointed to the whole abdomen, saying, "It's right there!" I tried to get him to be more specific, doing further exam in each groin and asking him about all the potential areas for hernia. He remained vague and got more and more agitated. I quietly excused myself so I could call his regular doctor and hopefully clarify the mystery.

As I was getting on the phone, Barb went back in to assist him. The next thing I saw through the glass partition separating us was him yelling and gesturing toward Barb. I'm sure I would have felt the same way no matter who was receiving the aggression, but in any case, that was my wife. The next thing I knew, I was standing almost nose to nose with him and we were shouting. There was a fair amount of adrenaline flowing and it was quite heated, to say the least. I told him I found his behavior unacceptable and that he was "fired" from being my patient. He said he was done with us anyway and rapidly left.

He was the only patient that I ever "fired." I was a little bigger than he was, but I was glad it didn't come to blows. The staff in the office were certainly glad to see him go and had been standing by ready to dial 911. They thought they had smelled alcohol on him.

I finally caught up with Tony's regular doctor. Still a little shaken, I explained what had happened. I could hear his smile through the phone. It turned out today was the man's last day of disability after being off work for a year. Apparently the hernia was his ticket to some more freedom. I never would have guessed that what started out as a search for a phantom hernia would lead to this outrageous incident at the office.

## Making a Difference

The patient, Beverly, was lying on the floor when I reached the room.

It was 2 AM. I was a surgery resident. The nurses called me because the patient had fainted. Several of the nurses were now assisting her quietly, but intensely. I noted immediately that she would lose consciousness when she would raise her head. Based on this alone, it appeared that she may have internal bleeding. When someone gets dizzy when they stand up, this can be a sign of *postural hypotension* (low blood pressure from not enough blood and/or fluids in their system). If she fainted just raising her head, things must be pretty bad.

I would come to learn later that Beverly was 45 years old. She was a lovely Southern Bell, with two teenage children. More importantly, she was in the hospital recovering from her liver transplant. This would be a big night for her.

The fifth-year resident soon appeared to give me a hand. We immediately began placing the IVs we typically insert in an emergency situation. Called *central line*, they are large IVs placed in the neck, shoulder, and groin where the large veins that are near the surface can be accessed.

We eventually placed four such lines. My chief even placed two of these in a single vein which I have never seen before or since. We gave IV fluids as fast as we could. I had learned by this point in my training to keep sending samples to the lab for analysis one after another in this type of emergency. I would send each lab every five to ten minutes and the results would take fifteen to twenty minutes to come back. This way I had a lot of data in process and "cooking" even before the first lab result came back.

The blood count (hemoglobin) was dropping rapidly. Ten, eight, six. Time to give blood. Time to go to surgery.

An old surgical principle became real for me that day. One big IV is better than multiple smaller ones. The openings in our multiple central lines were small. We were having trouble getting her enough IV fluids to sustain her.

In any case, we headed for the operating room.

The attending surgeon was standing in the hall. He was holding a cup of coffee and seemed tired. He asked, "Are you sure we need to take her down to surgery?" We had our hands full and kept on moving, essentially ignoring him. We quickly placed her on the operating room table.

Now it was the nurse who said she wasn't prepared for surgery. She needed to "count" before we could begin (prepare and count all the instruments, done at the beginning and end of a case, time allowing). She wasn't used to the "trauma" pace, being accustomed to a more leisurely elective setting.

We kept on working. This nurse seemed annoyed that we didn't follow her protocol. In the end, we mostly worked around her. We quickly covered the abdomen with disinfectant and took out the stitches. We cleaned up all the blood in the belly.

Beverly had ruptured the hookup of her liver artery. We repaired the leak and stabilized her.

She went on to survive, but she did require a new liver transplant. I carry a mental image of her hugging her children and again returning to work at the checkout at Walmart somewhere in the South.

*****

As surgical trainees, we didn't expect to get much recognition. I came to understand later on that goes with being a surgeon. It's a given that the stakes are high. You have great, glorious wins. You have devastating, personal losses. Some proportion of those wins and losses can be clearly attributed to your actions or your judgment, but over time you learn to do your best work while accepting that some factors are beyond your control. You can get stuck on congratulating or degrading yourself too heavily in the thick of that war.

After participating in stabilizing the patient, the head of the transplant program asked me to come to his office. He asked my name and we chatted briefly. Somewhere in that conversation, he mentioned that I had made a difference in this situation. I didn't get much more feedback than that, but it was a treasured moment. Surgery and surgical training are hard work, and it was gratifying to be recognized for making a difference.

---

*A neurosurgeon came into a busy nurses' station one day and announced "I'm here to operate on the baby!" He then went to put down his coffee and missed the counter by about 1 foot. It landed on the floor and splattered to the ceiling. You could "hear" everyone thinking, "Not on my baby, you're not!"*

# Surgery Isn't Hard To Do

Getting approval to perform surgical cases can be a politically charged issue. As one famous surgeon told me, "Surgery isn't hard to do. It's hard to *get to do.*"

I was working at a new hospital. I wanted to do a *laparoscopic adrenalectomy* (removal of a small tumor on the adrenal gland that rests on top of the kidney using several small incisions and a TV camera). The head of the Department of Surgery "denied me the privilege," claiming that I did not have enough experience.

A case like this was a rarity. I was an advanced laparoscopic surgeon and had a good record everywhere else that I had worked. I knew I deserved the right to do this case, but I was the new kid on the block and was subject to his decision.

I came back on a Monday morning after vacation time and was told that the case was ready to go. I was a little baffled in that the last I had heard I would not be able to do the case. I was told that everything had been approved including an okay from all the departments and the surgery department. I asked very specific questions about this and everything seemed to be in order. I immediately went up to the charge nurse in the operating room, who is the appropriate point person, and she acknowledged that I could proceed to do the case that morning. The patient was there and everyone was ready to go. I was pretty excited.

The patient and I reviewed all the details of surgery and she was ready to go. We brought her down to the room and the anesthesia was started.

On my way to the operating room, I happened to walk past the head of the Department of Surgery, who asked me what I was doing.

"The adrenal," I answered.

"But I didn't give you the privilege!" he quipped, and immediately left to find the head administrator.

The next thing I knew, the head of the hospital and he were shouting at each other in the hall. She (the head administrator) was dressed in street clothes in the middle of the operating room corridor (I hadn't seen that before!). They were literally yelling at each other, each one claiming that they had the final decision power. The argument was not settled regarding their powers, but it was decided that I should go ahead with this case in light of the fact that the patient was already prepared for surgery.

I was confident, but still this was a reasonably tricky surgery. Heaven forbid something should go wrong now, because there would be plenty of ammo to "crucify me." Unfortunately Shirley, the patient, weighed about 300 pounds, which complicated the situation.

It reminded me of the time when I told my senior partner about a patient who had threatened me if something went wrong during the surgery. My partner had replied, "It's a good thing you are a good surgeon."

In any case, we proceeded with Shirley's adrenal surgery. She did very well, and left the next day from the hospital feeling quite comfortable and happy that her surgery was over. The Chief of Surgery, however, accused me of doing surgery without privileges.

So I was asked to attend a large meeting where a decision would be made regarding the matter. At the appropriate time, I was called into the room. I said "hello" to the person I would be sitting next to at this meeting. I was seated at the end of two long rows of tables. Apparently on one side were the people on my side in the battle and on the other side were people who were against me. As I was new at the hospital, I hardly knew any of them.

Accusations started to fly. From one side of the room came something like, "Do you always do surgery without privileges at all the hospitals you go to?" The other side of the room jumped up and thumped on the tables, screaming "This is not a witchhunt!"

That went on for a while, and then suddenly it was decided that apparently I was okay. It was kind of weird feeling. They all got up and left and I was still there sitting alone in the room. I had never said anything but "hello" to the person sitting next to me. I didn't exactly feel welcome at this new hospital.

Interestingly enough, when my own work situation was changing, this same Chief of Surgery "asked me out to breakfast." We met at the hospital cafeteria, where I bought my own breakfast and we sat down to talk. I was a little mystified about what he could want from me. He then proceeded to make me a job offer to become an associate with him. It seemed ironic to me that he could dislike me so much before, and now be inviting me to work with him. The whole scene was strange, and I felt that he could have at least bought me a nice meal as part of the proceedings. Like the guy once said when I had him bent over the proctoscopy table, "You didn't even buy me lunch first."

In any case, I smiled and politely declined the offer to become his partner, then dismissed myself.

\*\*\*\*\*

The surgeon who said, "Surgery isn't hard to do, it's just hard to *get to do*" was Dr. Judson Randolph. He had written the core textbook in Pediatric Surgery. I worked with him as a third-year resident during a two-month rotation at Children's Hospital in Washington DC. One day on my rotation, there was a surgery case to change a hermaphrodite (half boy half girl) into a girl. The fellows and Chief Resident had planned to do the surgery. They were all tied up with other emergencies, so I was left alone to do the case with Dr. Randolph. This was frustrating to the rest of the team, who were quite envious.

It turned out that Dr. Randolph didn't scrub in. I ended up doing the surgery under his watchful eye. I was on a seat working on her bottom. He was leaning over with his head next to mine. That was when he told me the line that I still remember. "Surgery isn't hard to do. It's hard to *get to do*."

> *I sometimes wish I could put a video camera on my shoulder. You can walk in one room and be the total hero (once in a while you are; most the time you just did your job) and walk in the next room and be the total goat (same thing; once in a while you deserve it, most of the time it was factors out of your control; their particular healing characteristics, working under poor or infected circumstances etc.). You learn to try to sort it out. Give yourself some credit, be sad when it's warranted, and give yourself a break.*

# King James Day

It was going to be King James day.

The name was already memorable to me because of the Bible. His real name was James King, but in medicine we use the last name first so often, that in my mind, his name was King (comma) James.

I had a call from his regular doctor as I was leaving for Christmas vacation. The patient had seen me for office consultation regarding his hernia in August of the same year. In August, the doctor told me that his EKG had been abnormal. He had subsequently had open-heart surgery. The doctor called back now to let me know the patient was ready for his hernia repair.

The office staff were already gone on their Christmas vacation. Several days later, I called them from home. I told them that if the patient wanted, he could have a surgery day for his hernia after I came back. Thursday after my return would be fine. He could see me in the office if he wanted to discuss the date or just pick a surgery day.

Vacation was over and I was back in the office. King James was on the schedule to be seen. His paperwork, however, said that he was here for a fistula (blood vessel surgery for dialysis). Interesting. I went and asked him how he was doing etc. and then asked if he wasn't supposed to be here for hernia repair.

"No, I need a fistula."

Had I remembered it all wrong? Fine. We discussed his issues for the fistula and talked about possible surgery days.

I went out and asked the office staff, "Wasn't he supposed to get a hernia? Didn't I arrange for that before I left for vacation?"

"Don't think so."

"No, wait! I think he is on the schedule. In fact, he's on the schedule in two days. For hernia!"

Hmmmm. Then one of them remembered that the doctor had sent his paperwork. We looked back and sure enough, it was another "King James," verified by his different birthday.

People sharing a name isn't that unusual, although it's more typically a John Smith or Joe Brown. It made me smile however, that King James would happen to show up within two days of having King James on the schedule. This is the very reason that there is a general rule that two pieces of identification are required before something definitive (like surgery) is done. If you pay attention, you'll find that we usually ask for some other identifying feature like your birthday or possibly a phone number before something gets done medically.

I put both King James on the OR schedule for the same day, knowing that the OR staff would get a chuckle and be mindful of two patients with the same name.

---

*If one or two reasonably talented doctors aren't able to figure out your problem, your chances of getting an answer start to go down dramatically.*

# The Fight for Life

Karen had already been sick for over a week when I got called.

She had been on several forms of adrenaline for over a week. Something was affecting her system and giving her low blood pressure. The source of the problem wasn't clear. She had developed some abdominal bloating and mild abdominal tenderness. I was called at the request of her regular physician to evaluate whether this was the source of the problem coming to the surface or simply a reaction to her strong medicines.

The medicines had affected Karen's thinking and she was too sick to offer much help. I went to her husband to discuss the grave nature of her predicament. Even if the source could be identified, it wasn't clear that she could withstand the surgery/therapy that might be required. She didn't look like a very good candidate for someone to just "take a look under the hood" (i.e., to do exploratory surgery). He didn't have much to say. I think he already understood the difficult position she was in.

She was about 60 years old, but looked younger. She was "from a nice part of town." She had some history of arthritis but otherwise seemed healthy. I would later come to appreciate that she was both beautiful and pleasant.

So my first job was to sort this out. In some sense, the easiest way to do this would be to have proof of a problem with the bowel. Probably the most common and easily accessible proof can be elicited by a regular x-ray. If we can see gas outside the bowel (usually above the liver), this should be adequate verification that surgery would be required. We first tried the x-ray on her side, then with her sitting up. We could not verify "free air."

The next most useful piece of information would be a CT scan, so I ordered it. The nurse countered that the patient was too sick to make the trip through the hospital to the CT scanner. I responded that if there is a chance I was going to consider surgery, then she could make a trip to the CT scanner. We would need a team and equipment in case her heart stopped. I encouraged them to rapidly collect the necessary personnel and stuff required. Off we went to CT.

It reminds me of the story once told me by the hospital administrator. Her previous job had been at a famous hospital. One of the most recognized surgeons in the world had just had open-heart surgery where she was working. She got a call that the doctor/patient had decided to take a walk down the street to get a donut. The nurses wanted permission to physically restrain and/or sedate him. The administrator recommended that they allow him to take the walk, but be prepared for any contingency. I had to smile at the image of this world-famous person walking in his hospital gown with his IV pole with a whole gaggle of people, carts, and equipment behind him, "prepared for any contingency," going down the street to get his donut.

Similarly, we took her down, adrenaline drips and all, with the team prepared for any emergency. The CT scan eventually confirmed a small amount of air had leaked from the intestine. In retrospect, I wondered if I had been more patient in intensive care, could we perhaps have caught this bubble on the x-ray? I have since learned to be more patient, as the books recommend, and attempt to wait a few minutes with the patient in the appropriate position before snapping the x-ray to give every possibility for the leak to make itself known.

So we went to surgery. The bowel overall did not look very good. One spot in particular however, was not alive and had a leak. We took the piece out and brought the bowel out on her side. She would wear a bag for the bowel contents until we could get her in better shape. She tolerated the surgery adequately. Her recovery was slow, but complete. She would survive and return to a long period of full recovery.

Of note, her pathology report on the piece of bowel we took out came back with vasculitis. With vasculitis, the body treats the blood vessels as though they are a foreign object. The immune system kicks in, and tries to reject the blood vessel tissue. This causes all sorts of problems which can be treated with medicines that calm down the immune system, such as steroids. This type of reaction would explain why, even though she looked like she had infection, no source of infection was ever identified until the bowel finally ruptured. The symptoms that seemed to indicate infection were the result of the body trying to reject the blood vessels (i.e., itself).

In retrospect, her arthritis was rheumatoid arthritis. Because of overlapping etiology, it is likely that the vasculitis was related to her rheumatoid arthritis. What seemed like a relatively innocuous problem on the surface was actually the disease process that would come pretty close to taking her life.

Karen survived one of the longest runs of IV forms of adrenaline that I've encountered. This is especially significant in how complete and long-lasting her recovery was. It was another reminder to me to never underestimate what a body system can tolerate and still recover.

I met Karen again 15 years later, when her husband had gallbladder surgery. She reminded me that back then she had been paralyzed from the waist down in the midst of all her problems. Her only "residual" now was a leg brace she wore for foot drop. She was still beautiful, gracious and happy. I was proud to have been part of her healing.

*Surgery makes everyone nervous.*
*Being a surgical patient makes ME nervous.*

# The Long Week

It looked like it was going to be a bladder perforation.

The anesthesiologist had noticed the slightest twinge of blood in the catheter that was draining the bladder. We tested the bladder, and it appeared that I had placed my *trocar* (pointed tube placed through the abdominal wall in laparoscopic surgery) through the bladder.

I was doing an appendix on a young girl. I would typically insert three tubes into the abdomen. A larger one was placed at the belly button where the appendix would be removed. A second one was in the lower abdomen on the left and a third one was typically at the bottom of the abdomen. We would usually put a catheter in the bladder so that it was drained and kept out-of-the-way. This helped prevent the third tube, or trocar, from going through the bladder.

It was approaching midnight. I called my urologist friend to come help me with the repair.

While he was on the way, I went searching for the parents. I found the father, but told him I would wait until his wife was available so that I could speak with them both. I learned that night that it's best to talk as soon as possible to whomever is available. Another hard-won lesson.

As expected, they were not happy about the problem of the bladder perforation in their daughter. I delivered the news as evenly as possible and went back to finish the work. The urologist and I lengthened the quarter inch incision to approximately one inch in order to repair the bladder. All difficulty aside, I was pleased we could complete the surgery with small incisions.

After surgery, it was necessary to leave in the catheter to drain the bladder for two weeks. The family was disappointed to find out that her recovery would be further delayed by these issues.

The following day, a difficult problem unfolded with a woman, Juanita, who was bleeding in her intestines. To determine the source of the bleeding, we usually recommended an endoscopy (to look in the intestines with a tube). She refused this test. She continued to bleed and emergency surgery was indicated. She had difficulties after removal of her large intestine and developed an essentially lethal combination of problems. The unfortunate set of conditions that presented in Juanita included a rare but very sensitive reaction to blood so that it was essentially impossible to give her blood products. In addition, she required steroids to treat the issues related to her blood reaction. She had trouble with postoperative infection. The steroids added to her difficulty healing and fighting infection. The stress on her system led to further bleeding in the intestines, including a stomach ulcer. The bleeding, infection, and inability to transfuse painted her in a difficult corner, and she did eventually die.

Of note, after some time I would be sued in relation to this colon surgery. I traveled to New Jersey with my lawyer to hear the testimony of the doctor who would be the expert witness against me. We took the deposition on his ranch/farm. We were in the barn on the second floor, overlooking the horse arena. There were several expensive Mercedes and fancy "suits" spread around his property. It did not appear that he operated very often anymore, and this was confirmed by his own testimony. He claimed that the case would not have had problems if he had done it. My lawyer and I were eventually able to work through all the issues and the case was dropped.

My senior partner had been a very busy surgeon. He was out of town when I was tackling these cases. I was working very hard and long hours at the time. On that Monday through Friday, I got home every night after midnight and typically started at 5 AM for the new day. I'll never forget coming home Saturday morning at about 3 AM. It's hard to explain, but I was too tired to sleep. I sat in a chair in the dark listening to Doobie Brothers' *South City Midnight Lady*. Sleep would finally come, but it took some time to contemplate what I'd just been through.

*****

The family of the girl with the bladder perforation lived nearby. A surgeon once told me, "Be careful about operating on your neighbor. If something happens, you may be stuck looking at them over the fence." Possibly true, but I take a slightly different view. I've often felt that you're better off with one reasonably talented local doctor who is personally interested in your case than a whole team of experts who might be there just to take care of their own small part.

Sometimes people ask my advice on whether they should get a surgeon "downtown" (at a larger medical center) or one near where they live for a relatively routine procedure. I suggest that a reasonably talented person in their neighborhood may at times have a more personal interest in their outcome. In some sense, the local guy might be a little more responsive to a problem than letting "the system" and/or "the team" take care of it.

*****

As it turned out, my urology friend was also a friend of the family whose daughter had the perforated bladder. I believe he talked to them on my behalf and may have helped comfort them in a way that I could not during this difficult time. Years later, I would learn that the girl's bladder had an anatomical variation. Apparently this was diagnosed at some point after my surgery and that was why my normal trocar placement caused bladder perforation. It was welcome news for me to find this out. Often there is more to a story that unfolds down the road and we rarely hear about it. In this case, learning these details cleared up a nagging question that had lingered in my mind.

# Hit the Road

It was going to be my first and only ambulance ride.

It was about 6 PM Saturday night on the holiday weekend shortly before Christmas and I was finishing up my work. I was putting in IVs at a ventilator hospital (a special hospital for people recovering from respiratory conditions). I was doing my best to get out of there, when the nurse asked if I would remove one more IV before I left. It was a larger IV, used for dialysis, and typically placed in a large vein. This particular catheter was near the top of the leg.

I cut the stitches and pulled the catheter.

Blood nearly hit the ceiling.

The nurses on this holiday evening and weekend shift didn't seem very interested in any excitement and quietly slipped away. I was left holding pressure on the area to see if I could stop the bleeding. Eventually the house manager came down and asked how things were going. I was grateful to see that at least she appeared to have an understanding of what was happening.

Instead of the vein, the catheter had been placed in the artery. Virtually next to each other, this was not necessarily an unusual mishap. I would come to find out later that the catheter had been placed by my associate, who had been working with us for a year.

In any case, I was standing with my hand in the groin controlling the bleeding. The house manager would stop by every half-hour or so and ask, "How's it going?"

I would take my hand off the area. We would both see the squirt of blood, and she would offer to check back again in a while. At about her fourth time back, she asked, "Call the ambulance?"

I checked once more. Still bleeding. "Yes please."

So I got my ride in the ambulance. Hand in groin, we loaded

the patient and ventilator into the ambulance. Sirens going, no stopping for red lights, it was about a 30 minute trip to the regular hospital. I had arranged for the vascular surgeon to meet me in the operating room. He had left his Christmas party and we all converged fully dressed, me with my hand in the groin, in the operating room. It felt like a rather large crowd (ambulance people, operating room nurses, nurses from the other hospital, vascular surgeon etc.) had gathered to watch as I slowly took my hand off the groin. The bleeding had stopped!

The vascular surgeon and I looked at each other. There was no chance we would risk a re-bleed after all that. We prepared her and did the surgery to put a stitch where the hole was in the artery.

We now have a device to hold pressure so that no one has to get caught and stand there in these situations. The classic "trick" was to ask someone standing nearby "could you hold pressure for a minute?" and then you could disappear for a while. In addition, we often use ultrasound now to place these IVs, so that IV placement is more precise. I'm thankful that we don't experience episodes like this as often anymore.

---

My thoughts on personal finance:
You always have 10% less than you need.

# The Assistant's Down

I was placing an IV in a larger shoulder vein on Norma, a hospitaized patient. It's called a *central line*. Although I don't need a lot of help, I generally have an assistant to hand me a few things and assist the patient. I called the desk and asked them to send someone down to help me.

The placement is a bit of a procedure. We position the patient lying flat on their back. We often tip the head of the bed down a little bit. We undress and sterilize the shoulder and numb up the area around the clavicle/shoulder bone. We then use a needle about 5 inches long to slide under the bone and find the vein.

My help had arrived. I asked her to come over and give me the flush solution. I had on my hat, mask, and sterile gloves. I had to help her get the right solution and hold it correctly. This didn't seem unusual with the wide variety of help and experience in the hospital. I asked her to hold the patient's hand. I took up the "big needle" after numbing the patient and started the procedure to find the vein. I looked up just in time to see the eyes of my helper rolling back in her head. I managed a running catch just before she hit the floor. I called the front desk and asked for more help. The nurses helped my assistant. They took her away and got things straightened out.

Fainting is not necessarily unusual around hospital work. We all know you have to keep a close eye on the dad watching his first C-section. My father-in-law, a surgeon, once fainted helping me with a colon resection in the early AM which gave the anesthesiologist two patients for a while. I routinely tell the new student nurses in the operating room to ask for help if they get that warm, lightheaded feeling. Patients will occasionally go down during a blood draw. I sometimes joke with the patients in the office who are concerned about fainting during a minor procedure. I tell them to go ahead and faint; then I won't have to numb them up.

In any case, I eventually learned that my helper for the central line was actually a hospital visitor. How she managed to get that far without straightening out our communication, I'll never know. I can only imagine the story she told her family at dinner that night.

> *When someone obstinately tells us we need to operate, we describe them as having the "bravado of the noncombatant."*

## Just Checking...

It was late. I was driving back to reoperate on an elderly gentleman.

Frederic's original problem was a cancer of the first portion of the small intestine. This is called the duodenum. On its own, this would be a tumor that is in a "high rent district" (i.e., many critical structures). In addition, however, he had difficulties in the past with polyps of the colon, near the other end of the intestine. He had had multiple benign tumors, or polyps, removed from the right colon. Some had only been partially removed and he needed this portion of bowel out as well. Overall, he required an extensive operation.

In my mind, Frederic truly was a gentleman. He had been an immigrant, but held himself quite stately. He was kind and gentle, and had a lovely wife with a beautiful smile. He was 86, lived in Canada and owned and operated his own factory there. I had to smile, because he liked to "winter" in Chicago. He was engaging and distinguished when he spoke. In our brief encounters, he would tell me stories of his travels, adventures, love, and the wars he had fought in.

We had finished his operation earlier that day. We had taken out both pieces of bowel and put them back together.

After surgery, he was having a relatively "rough landing." His blood pressure was intermittently low, requiring IV doses of forms of adrenaline. He was not making much urine, and had some evidence of partial kidney shutdown. His abdomen was extremely tender, with pain that seemed out of proportion to his large but fairly soft belly.

His repeat CT scan was not diagnostic of any particular

problem. Postop changes were noted on the CT, including expected *postoperative rearrangement of the intestines.*

Post operative rearrangement of the intestines.

I considered this. The bowel has natural twists in the abdomen from before birth that keep it pinned down and therefore not vulnerable to twisting. There are some syndromes where these "twists" are incomplete and the bowel is insufficiently pinned down. In these cases, at some point in a person's life, the bowel can twist on its base. This base holds all the blood vessels to the intestines. When it twists, the bowel loses its blood supply and starts to die. If you don't address this immediately, people lose essentially all of their small intestine. It's a disaster.

So I considered his "postoperative rearrangement of the intestines." This particular combination of removing a piece of bowel at the top end of the intestines and taking out a piece of colon had placed the small bowel down the right side of the abdomen and the colon in the left side of the abdomen. In some sense I had potentially re-created the "untwisted" bowel which could be susceptible to rotation and all the subsequent problems.

Even though the bowel had been placed back carefully at surgery, I had to consider this possibility. I broke into a cold sweat. I have distinctly come to hate this feeling when I'm cold and hot, prickly and sweaty all over my body all at the same time.

This would be one of those times.

This would also be one of those times when the best and possibly only answer would come from another surgery. To merely observe a patient has a potential for disaster. Other fancy testing might be possible, but it could burn up precious moments. It was certainly possible, if not probable, that his combination of issues were all simply postoperative problems that would correct themselves given time. With the magnitude of the potential disaster, however, the risk-benefit ratio would clearly be on the side of reoperation. It turns out, in reality, that going back into surgery, while it may be nearly the ultimate nuisance, is a very low risk to someone in the case of a "negative laparotomy" (when we open the abdomen to look for any problems, but do not find anything wrong).

So I talked with the patient and family, and we went back to surgery.

I told the nurses as we prepped that I would know in about two seconds after the first stitches were out whether our night would be long or short. Worse yet, potentially, the longer my night, the shorter his life. I took out the staples and popped the stitch and saw pink bowel. I could have kissed it. I paused for the briefest, undetectable second to give a little prayer of thanks. I would later do a happy dance in the hall on the way out.

We took this opportunity to double-check the abdomen. I put in a couple of extra stitches so that I would avoid another episode of cold sweat on his behalf. We closed the incision and Frederic began his otherwise unremarkable recovery.

Frederic got a firsthand understanding of why "you never want to be an interesting case."

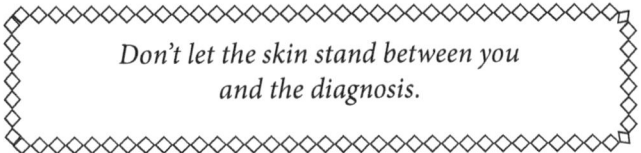

*Don't let the skin stand between you and the diagnosis.*

# Not Social Anymore

It was a hard one for me to figure out as a medical student.

The attending had admitted the patient, Felix, to the hospital and told me to go check him out. He was about 50 years old. Overall, he seemed okay to me. No pain, answering my questions, no apparent mental or physical discomfort.

I continued the discussion with his wife, who felt that he was somehow different as of late.

"He isn't as social," was her comment.

I was quite thorough in my physical examination in those days. I'm pretty sure that I cannot repeat that now in the same fashion.

The only thing unusual was the back of his eyes. I noticed when looking with the ophthalmoscope that there appeared to be some swelling. I'm sure this would be obvious to an eye doctor, but I had never seen it before. In spite of the potential dire consequences of this finding for the patient, I was excited that I had recognized it.

The attending asked what I would like to do next.

"CT scan," I said.

"Order it, and let me know," came the reply.

We soon had the result. The CT scan showed a fairly large cancer in the frontal lobe portion of the brain.

As with other areas of the body, a tumor in this area can advance fairly significantly before being detected. In retrospect, the mental status changes that his wife noted and the *papilledema* that I discovered, although subtle on a larger scale, were consistent with the final diagnosis that would reveal itself.

Still, for me, as I worked through the problem in real time, it was fascinating to see it unfold. Losing your social interest just didn't seem like enough of a problem to end up with the diagnosis that he had.

As an interesting side note, I think this case may have been crucial to my winning an internal medicine award for my medical school class. I had been counseled that, since I would practice surgery for the rest of my life, it would benefit me to pursue as many nonsurgical/internal medicine rotations as possible as a medical student. I'm sure this helped me earn the award, but it turned out this advice did not serve me well when I finally started surgical rotations because I had some serious catching up to do.

In any case, I got the award, and I know I'm drawing on this aspect of my training whenever I'm able to put subtle findings together into a diagnosis.

> *We often have to make significant or dramatic decisions based on limited information. Making the right diagnosis is often the hard part, as opposed to knowing what to do once the diagnosis is made. Sometimes I tell people, "I wish the universe would shoot out a little card with the correct diagnosis for me, because I would know exactly what to do." When I'm discussing the plan for a patient who doesn't need surgery at that moment, I tell the residents, "We have a plan. That's the most important part."*

# The Long Road to Life

So many unforgettable things took place during residency.

It was a snowy day when Anita came into our trauma service. We would find out later how the accident happened. She apparently had car trouble on the highway. In the course of events, she was straddling the guard rail. A larger cargo truck had slipped in the snow, falling onto its side. Apparently, as it was sliding along the guard rail it caught her, smashing her leg and dragging her along. She weighed about 500 pounds.

So we started to sort out the injuries. She had terrible cuts on her "bottom" where the guard rail had ripped her. They went up to the bone both in the front and the back. The skin on the leg that had gotten caught between the rail and the truck was only attached at the ankle and at the buttock. You could take the skin anywhere along the leg and it would essentially move freely without attachment from the top to the bottom. The only visual hint of the disaster was a small hole in the skin near the ankle where dissolved fatty tissue was coming out. Otherwise, if she was just lying flat, the leg looked essentially normal.

We had put in the breathing tube and were checking her vitals intermittently with the Doppler (a blood flow test and pulse monitor that makes the characteristic "whoosh whoosh" sound). We noted we would get a pulse of a hundred and forty whenever the Doppler was being used down near the groin or lower abdomen, which did not match her wrist pulse of a hundred and ten.

We were perplexed about this, but the mystery was solved when the abdominal x-ray came back. She had a baby on board! We were intermittently obtaining the baby's pulse instead of the mother's pulse.

Immediately, we realized that she could not deliver this baby naturally with the terrible tears on her bottom. It was pretty rare that the obstetricians were involved in our traumas, but it was obvious that a C-section would be required. They came down, and we helped them do the C-section on this heavier lady. Fortunately, a healthy child was delivered.

We then resumed the trauma work that was ahead of us. We placed the colostomy (a bag on her side to drain on her stool) and stitched up all the tears on her bottom. On the injured leg, we then removed all the skin that was not going to survive. We attempted to harvest the skin and reapply skin grafts to her at that time. With all her other issues, this initially did not take well, but eventually we were able to get coverage with skin grafts and other surgeries, etc.

Anita stabilized and survived. Interestingly enough, she was not aware that she was pregnant when the injuries occurred. I'm sure she was more surprised than we were when she got the outcome of that day.

*****

Anita came back to visit us quite often after she was healed. In fact, I learned from nurses who worked there after I left that she continued to come for years afterwards. She usually came on the anniversary date of the original accident. This had become a turning point in her life. She lost weight, got an education and a job. The son, Henry, who surprised her and us, would accompany her for the visits.

> *I once operated on a nationally known comedian. I prayed that I would not be featured in one of her acts..*

# The Other Side of Pain

Lawsuits are very personal to us as physicians. We want the best outcome possible for our patients. It goes without saying that when there's a lawsuit, something has interfered with attaining this outcome.

I once met a surgeon who had lost a lawsuit. He shared some of the aspects of the case with me. He felt he had performed an appropriate surgery. The patient had a poor outcome and developed a chronic condition postoperatively. Her disability was apparently evident during the lawsuit proceedings.

The surgeon lost the suit for a significant amount beyond his malpractice coverage. He was a wreck. He had been looking ahead to retirement soon. I felt for him as he turned over his personal money and possessions.

It's safe to say it changed me. I can't say it made me change how I do my job, because I always felt I did the best job I could. But it made me more wary and uneasy, feeling like I need to look over my shoulder all the time.

I also felt sad because he seemed to me to be a talented surgeon and a caring person. He was well respected in his community. His experience left me with lingering questions about the fairness of the legal system.

I understand the need for people to be compensated for a loss. I agree they are entitled to their day in court for true malpractice. However, the difference between a bad outcome and malpractice can sometimes be a fine line.

The current legal system can process a lawsuit with some level of variability. Sometimes it seems like the same case could be malpractice one time and a poor outcome another time, depending on the judge, lawyer, jury, injury, records and so forth. In a perfect world, if we could trust that everyone really had done "the right thing" during a surgical procedure, one of my wishes would be a pool set up for people who experience a bad outcome after surgery or who had something unpredictable occur in relation to the surgery. They would be entitled to an award in recognition of the fact that the outcome was not what anyone would have expected, but the process would be more "no-fault." The way it stands now, the payment/award can seem somewhat arbitrary.

The court proceedings themselves can feel very personal. A surgeon friend of mine was so distracted by the things he had been accused of during court that he wrecked his car on the way home after the trial. Surgeons who have been sued know the feeling of being examined microscopically under an intense barrage of accusations. Sometimes it feels like it might take more strength to stand up under this kind of pressure than it does to work through a fourteen hour day of dealing with very sick patients.

My heart goes out to everyone who has had a less than perfect outcome after surgery. It is not the surgeon who has to live with these (often permanent) results, but the sadness is felt by all parties. Surgery is an intense experience for everyone involved. It's not surprising that the intensity of the experience continues in any legal proceedings that may follow.

*You can make a bad impression in a day.*
*It can take you years to make a good one.*

# Call Again

Surgery can be a winding road.

The first call came before midnight. Alex was a 75-year-old social worker in the emergency room. He was there with his wife. The scan had shown "free air," indicating a piece of bowel was leaking. The gas, however, was minimal, the patient was only mildly tender and was quite stable. The usual rule if the colon is leaking is to take out that area and create a colostomy (pull a piece of the intestine through the skin with a bag installed on the person's side where the stool would drain).

In his case, however, it might be possible to "pull a rabbit out of a hat" and give him a brief bowel prep, take a piece out and put him back together in one sitting. This would be pushing the surgical envelope a little bit, but would clearly have an advantage for the patient. The emergency room doctor said, "Both the patient and wife have a lot of questions. You can discuss it with them."

The next call was at approximately 12:30 AM. Another ER doctor with another patient, Anastacia. This patient had right sided pain and gallstones. The rest of the story seemed fairly unremarkable. She would be admitted and I could offer her surgery in the morning. Thanks for the call.

The next call came at approximately 1:00 AM. Alex, the "free air" patient preferred another hospital. He would be transferred. Thanks for the call.

It was 1:30 AM and the phone rang again. They had decided to do a CT scan on Anastacia, the gallbladder lady. The CT now showed appendicitis and a kidney mass. A gallbladder is a morning case. An appendectomy is sometimes a "get out of bed case." Her pain had been about the same for these two months. Her white count/blood count did not indicate infection and her pain was not dramatic. So I made the decision to wait a few more hours until morning. It seemed reasonable to deal with it then.

An uncle of mine once told me he met a neurosurgeon that he liked. He had gone to see the surgeon for an opinion about neck surgery. It was apparently a difficult determination, but the neurosurgeon ultimately recommended nonsurgical treatment. The neurosurgeon had made an interesting comment, noting, "It took me six months to learn how to do neurosurgery and four and a half years to learn when." I hoped that my surgical judgment would not betray me on this night.

So I got up early and went to see the gallbladder/appendix/kidney mass lady. I reviewed her CT scan, then reviewed it again with the radiologist. It appeared most consistent with a kidney cancer. There was some local swelling, and it appeared to me that the appendix was caught in the swelling. The radiologist, however, said that there was a reasonable if not high likelihood that this was appendicitis. There were gallstones; however, the gallbladder was unremarkable. I was grateful the ER doc had pursued the CT scan.

Well, on the scale of surgical triage, appendicitis wins in this situation. I couldn't honestly tell if there was appendicitis or not, but I wouldn't be able to defend myself if it were written in the report and I did not respond to it. So, the kidney mass/cancer would have to wait until the acute issues were dealt with. I called the urologist to verify this and he agreed.

I walked up to check in with the patient. I asked, "What have you been told about this?" She appeared to be about 55, well kept, and mildly nervous about being in the hospital.

"Appendicitis," she said.

I paused a minute, then said, "We need to talk."

I could see a shadow pass across her face. I gently explained about the kidney mass and the significant probability of cancer. It's always a little harder when the patient has started down a certain path of expectation and you find that something more serious is going on. We worked through the issues and implications. We started waking up family members by phone to discuss this with them as well. It would be a long discussion with lots of questions for which, at that point, I would have few clear answers. Most imminently, however, she still needed the appendix out. So we discussed this as well. She agreed and I made the arrangements.

As the final chapter in her winding road, the appendix was in fact caught in the swelling of the kidney mass. I could not do the surgery laparoscopically and I needed to make an incision to get the job done. Ironically, even though she didn't have appendicitis, the surgery was more challenging than average because the swelling made the entire area difficult to deal with. We managed. I got the appendix out, and then worried afterwards for a few days that there might be further complications. She eventually recovered and went home to prepare for her next surgery involving the kidney.

Another surgery hero, she recovered her composure and prepared for the next fight that would be required as she tackled the kidney cancer. Who would have guessed that her "gallbladder" turned appendix would turn out to be kidney cancer.

> *I once did a cancer surgery on a friend of mine. I asked him if he felt differently about himself after the journey of cancer. He commented that sometimes, when he's riding his motorcycle, he wonders if there will be a goat or flock of birds on the road around the next corner that will kill him. To him, facing this experience was just another possible "goat on the road."*

# No Vitals

"It's a gunshot to the head. The patient has no vitals." This was the report we received on the trauma unit.

I was a second year resident spending time on the trauma service. This was one of the best venues for residents to get lots of practice and we learned to expect the unexpected.

The patients at this old hospital would come to the emergency room. If it was considered a "trauma," the patient would be triaged to our trauma unit on the third floor. Occasionally we would get a phone call alerting us that something unusual would be coming up. Today's special patient would be a gunshot to the head.

We cleared the area and set up surgical trays in case there was a chance to salvage. The door swung open and a woman sitting on a cart was pushed into the area.

"Get her out of the way! We have a gunshot to the head coming," we urged, to keep the area clear.

We placed her in the back corner and continued to wait.

A few minutes later, she quietly said, "I was shot in the head."

We all turned to look at her, then walked over to see what she was talking about.

Sure enough, there was a bullet hole in the back of her scalp. We did an x-ray. The bullet had splayed out under her scalp. No therapy was required. We cleaned the wound and discharged her.

We checked back with the emergency room about this patient. "No vitals?"

"We didn't take any vitals."

She had vitals, they just hadn't taken them!

With this play on words, this woman had gone from being virtually dead in our minds to discharged without treatment.

Bless her.

# Margaritaville and the Mudder Horse

One time my wife Barb and I went to Las Vegas for a couple days with some other couples. I had been in practice working now for about 15 years.

I really like Jimmy Buffett. I wanted to go to his bar *Margaritaville* in Las Vegas, but I couldn't get anyone to go with me. I finally let Barb know I would be gone for a couple hours in the afternoon to check it out.

"Yeah, sure. Go for it!" (She's helped me get to several other Buffet places, including "the original" *Cheeseburger in Paradise* restaurant in Florida, bless her heart.)

I drove from the hotel down to the strip. It was a beautiful sunny afternoon, probably about 70°. I took a seat at the second-floor bar with my back to the sun. I was looking at the *shot six holes in my freezer* freezer. I didn't really feel like I needed to talk to anyone. The bartender seemed nice enough. A "cheeseburger in Paradise" and a drink or two and I would be on my way (I'm not really a daytime drinker).

It turned out that the Kentucky Derby was later that afternoon.

I was sitting next to a regular looking guy who appeared to be about my age, and he wanted to chat a little. Turns out, he used to lead weeklong hunting trips on horseback in Wyoming. I mentioned, when he asked my occupation, that I was a surgeon. We chatted a little more.

In an attempt to make conversation, I prodded him, "You must get some unique people. How was it taking people on the trips?"

He talked a little about some of his experiences, then added, "But the surgeons were the worst. They would always tell me where to go to get the best hunting. I'd been tracking down animals to hunt for 40 years in those hills. But I didn't know enough about it to help *them*! I eventually gave up trying to convince them of this and I finally just went where they wanted. Cost me a few dry hunting trips."

Ouch?!? As my "first lesson" that day, his comments rang true in a personal way. Just because you're good at one thing doesn't mean you're good at everything. It's an easy mistake for surgeons to make. You've got to have enough ego to do your job, but it tends to spill over into life.

It reminded me of the time when I came home during my chief resident year in training. At the time, I was responsible for a group of approximately 15 people, including medical students and residents. We ran a busy surgery service, and I was responsible for coordinating them. Sometimes we did 15 to 20 surgeries a day and I'd make sure things ran smoothly. Needless to say, I got used to being in charge and "barking orders."

So I came home after one of those days, and apparently I was still "barking orders." Barb gently looked at me and said, "No, you're home now. *You* take out the garbage."

This was just one of many lessons that helped me to distinguish between what I do well and what I just imagine I do well! I've become more comfortable with the multiple roles we have to play in life.

*****

Which leads me to my second eventual lesson of the day:

So this fellow and I continued talking about surgery. He related how, on one of the hunting trips, he met the woman who was to become his wife. And it turns out she's a general surgeon.

And then he went on to share with me about what it's like to live with a general surgeon. By his description, it gave new meaning to "high maintenance." Not in a "it takes a lot of money" or there are "high expectations for living standards" kind of way. But a general surgeon endures a high level of stress, and because of that, they need a fair amount of space and understanding. He mentioned that it was not uncommon for his wife to come home and not be conversant. She would go to a secluded place in the house until she recovered enough to be social. This might sometimes take a few hours. He, meanwhile, would try various things to help smooth the way, like putting together a nice candlelight dinner or whatever other provisions he could organize. He seemed to have a good grasp of the fact that her work was challenging in ways he couldn't even imagine and that he could play an important part by not adding to the stress.

But my take-home message wasn't to expect someone else to take care of my stress. It was an acknowledgment that I had a job that could make me a little tough on people. It kindled a renewed desire in me to find ways to manage my own stress so I could be a better friend, partner, person. Barb has helped me a lot with this journey.

Somehow during the conversation, my friend at the bar gave me the sense that being a cowboy had helped prepare him for his role as support person to his wife. If I'm not mistaken, he alluded to being patient with livestock that might be having an off day...

Eventually the conversation moved on to the Kentucky Derby. It had been raining in Kentucky that day. Someone at the bar mentioned that such and such horse was "a good *mudder*." Apparently, a mudder is a horse that runs well under messy conditions. I double-checked the name of the horse and separated myself from the conversation so I could place my bet. I shook hands with my new friend Derk and took off for our hotel.

I had never placed a bet on a horse. I assumed it took some special language, but I had no idea what this was. One of our friends was supposed to meet me near the place to bet. It was very crowded, with everyone looking at the screens getting ready for the big race. I couldn't find him. I even tried to call him. No answer.

As it got close to race time, I decided I had to make my move. I went up to the betting window and asked in plain language to put 20 bucks (I was out of control!) on my newly found mudder horse to win. I wasn't sure I said it right, because several of them stared at me funny. But I got the ticket.

I didn't even have time to get back to where my friends were gathered. The race was off.

And my mudder horse won! 9 to 1 odds to boot!

I was thrilled! I went to my friends and told them how excited I was that I had won. The group got really quiet. Apparently they had been researching and researching this race, and I was the only one in the end who won. I kept the rest of my celebration to myself.

My payout was $180. Of course, in Vegas, the hundred dollar portion came as a single hundred dollar bill. I don't get many of those. I kept the hundred dollar bill in my wallet for a long time, thinking of my lessons from Margaritaville and my mudder horse.

---

*A good friend once told me "My doctor is like my bookie. He just gives me the odds for all the possibilities."*

## Joy of Surgery

Sometimes you forget just how amazing it is that a body can heal itself after surgery and that you're not really the healer. If your body cannot heal itself, the surgeon will have to deal with the consequences. You learn this quickly when someone has a compromised immune system (from chemotherapy, AIDS, etc.) or has a blood-clotting disorder. Still, it's a privilege to go in and "rearrange the pieces" and leave it so someone with healing capabilities can actually be better off.

Aaron was a patient in his 40s (which now seems young to me). He had a groin hernia that was at least fist size. He ran a little carpentry business locally. He didn't have any insurance. The hernia was keeping him from riding his bike to work.

I can almost always work out an agreeable payment plan. The hospital, however, will not negotiate. In addition, for someone with no insurance, they expect the money in advance. On top of that, they often require the inflated charge rate, not the average ("discounted?!?") insurance rate.

I had recently joined a local surgery center, and they had a rule that required us to do two procedures a year for free. This apparently fulfilled their "charity" obligations to the state. Neither the surgeon nor the surgery center could charge the patient. I was happy to be able to offer this service to Aaron and he was delighted to accept this opportunity.

It was a strange feeling going in to do the hernia on the prearranged day. Maybe it was just the day, but I felt like I was getting to do surgery just for the pure joy of it. Somehow doing the service for free released me from the financial obligations that surround each case. To me, it felt like surgery for the joy of surgery. I felt relaxed, and simply enjoyed the beauty and privilege of the dissection, the anatomy, the wonders of anesthesia, and the fun and fulfillment of fixing a problem. It was a unique feeling that stayed with me for a while.

The government's position regarding the "self-pay" patient sometimes mystifies me. One of the basic rules in this regard states that you have to treat any patient that comes into your emergency room. The government makes this rule, but makes no provision who will pay As surgeons, we are required to take this ER call for the hospital where we work. In fact, not only will we not be paid, but we carry the overhead (malpractice insurance, office expense etc.). This is somewhere in the range of $200-$300 for every patient in my practice. It does seem that surgeon pay used to be such that charity would be automatically included and expected. I can see potential for this to be the case less and less in the future, as surgeon pay declines.

The other interesting outcome, it seems, is the undue stress that this position places on hospitals in economically challenged neighborhoods. The hospitals with minimal "self-pay" population tend to look like hotels. The hospitals with a lot of "self-pay" can barely stay in business.

I personally don't find that most self-pay patients are in that situation by their choice. When I hear about their circumstances, I think they're just too poor to afford insurance.

In a perfect world, from my surgeon standpoint, it would be nice if there was a law requiring health insurance. I can't even begin to fathom the politics involved in that statement. I just find it interesting that car insurance can be required in my state but not health insurance. Another law that I would consider if I could put all implications aside, would be that insurance companies must take all comers. As long as they can pick their customers, the bottom line leads them to accept only healthy people. Taking all comers would require them to price the insurance for the population and not just for the healthy segment that they can choose.

Altogether, I think physicians typically appreciate their unique ability to help someone who is sick regardless of their ability to pay. I don't always think about the wonder of surgery when I do a case for free, but I do think I carry a sense of the importance of restoring health to that individual.

I am currently blessed to work for a hospital that supports the doctors in caring for the poor. In a system that sometimes seems patched together, I'm grateful for a hospital that's willing to stand in the gap.

---

*Don't tick off your surgeon right before he is going to operate on you.*

# Expert help

I received the call from the emergency room. They were concerned that the patient, Janna, had a flesh eating infection. She had come in with blisters on her hand. Over her several hours in the emergency room, the eruption had traveled up her forearm and was now just above her elbow.

If true, she had a potentially serious problem. Several bacteria can work together, and literally eat the tissue as they go. The tissue that is left behind is dead. In principle, the only cure is to cut out the bad tissue ahead of the infection. If it gets somewhere where you can't cut around it, the patient dies.

I went in to the hospital immediately. I had also called in the operating room team. I suspected they were right. If it were true, it looked like we would have to remove her arm.

I had not done this before. I asked that the orthopedic surgeon on call that night assist me. It was arranged.

As I was heading toward the operating room area, I saw one of the junior orthopedic surgery attendings coming down the hall. She was carrying a big stack of books under her arms. I assumed that this was the person called in to give me help with this case.

"I'm so glad I got called. I've never seen this surgery before," she said.

Hmmmmm. So much for someone who could give me some guidance.

We took Janna to surgery. I made several incisions in the forearm and confirmed that the tissue was dead. By now the blisters were on her shoulder. We made the incision to take off her arm, leaving enough skin to get the area closed. We could see that the infection and dead tissue was just getting to the area leading into the chest. If the infection went into her skull or inside her chest, we would not be able to help her. We got there just in time. We took off her arm, put in the drains, and stitched her up.

In the end, it wasn't very hard. We just had to find the blood vessels and tie them off. We both learned that night how to do a "fore quarter" amputation (arm amputation).

Unfortunately for Janna, she was also a dialysis patient. Not only did she lose an arm, but she also lost a place where she could get her ongoing dialysis treatments. I suppose it's a tough example of the phrase "adding insult to injury."

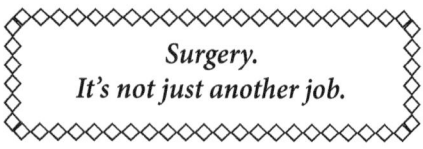

*Surgery.*
*It's not just another job.*

# Falling Scalpel

We were first-year residents in surgery training when it happened.

There were about six of us at the time. One of the residents, George, was operating with the head of our program. As you might imagine, operating with the head of the program was stressful for us. For instance, the head surgeon was known to take away the operating room suction device from the resident and give it to the medical student, who was lower on the totem pole. The resident would then have to stand there without doing anything. It didn't help our training and was belittling as well.

So George was in operating with "the boss." The boss laid the scalpel on the patient's chest. The patient was lying flat on the operating room table, and the scalpel slid off the patient and fell to the floor.

But the scalpel didn't make it to the floor. The scalpel blade made a direct landing right into George's shoe.

The room got very quiet, and everyone looked down at George's shoe.

George gritted his teeth and said, "Just pull the knife out, pour some Betadine on my shoe, and keep operating." So the nurse did this.

The boss was particularly sensitive to people being stuck. He had been stuck by a resident once himself and had contracted hepatitis. This eventually became a life-threatening issue for him.

The boss was normally quite outspoken during surgery. He became fairly quiet for the rest of this case. In fact, for the next five years of training, he didn't bother George at all.

So, we were all at a party in the final year of training five years later, when someone brought up the story of the knife in

George's shoe. George was standing nearby, and a sly smile spread across his face. He 'fessed up.

The scalpel had actually never hit him when it struck his foot. It had dropped between his toes. His quick thinking response made everyone think he had been cut. The final significance of that event was not an injury, but a "get out of jail free card" from the boss.

> *As a surgeon, it's not my job to tell you what to do. It's my job to give you enough information to make an informed decision. Then, if you need surgery and opt for it, I would be glad to be the one to help you.*

# Appendix Once and for All

The call came at an awkward time.

My family and I were heading toward downtown to watch fireworks on the Fourth of July. The traffic on Lakeshore Drive had just come to a complete stop, about 1 mile from our actual destination. We were now in a parking lot. The cars were bumper-to-bumper, four lanes wide.

The call came from the emergency room. They had an 11-year-old boy, Sam, who looked like he had appendicitis. The CT scan findings, however, were somewhat vague, not absolutely confirmatory. I told them where I was, and that I expected I would be free at about midnight to come and evaluate the patient. They said Sam was stable; they were not excited about the delay, but said that it should work out okay.

The ER doctor seemed mildly uncomfortable, though, and eventually said that the dad wanted to talk to me. The father asked what my plan was, and I explained to him that there would be some delay, but that upon my arrival I would evaluate his son to consider an appendectomy. The father said he didn't really want an evaluation. He just wanted the appendix taken out.

"Okay," I said. "Once I get there, we'll make sure that it looks like appendicitis and we'll get things going." He again said he just wanted the appendix removed.

I repeated again what I thought was kind of obvious, "I'll take a look and we'll figure it out."

"No, you don't understand," he went on. "I've had him into the ER four or five times. Each time there's a delay until you guys get here. When the surgeon comes, he says there's no pain or it doesn't look like appendicitis anymore, and the job doesn't get done. I don't really care what you think, I just want his appendix out. I have five other kids; I can't keep taking this one to the emergency room."

I considered this for a minute, standing outside my car in the warm July evening in the newly formed parking lot. Not all that unreasonable, after all.

"All right," I said. "As soon as I get my car moving again, I'll come there and take his appendix out." He seemed relieved.

We watched the fireworks sitting on our car on Lakeshore Drive. When it was over, I dropped the family off and went to the hospital. Just as in the dad's prior experiences, Sam was pain free. The CT scan was not diagnostic. True to my word, we took him up in the middle of the night and removed his appendix. It didn't look that bad to me, and was probably normal. Sam recovered uneventfully and went home.

A surgeon friend of mine had a somewhat similar experience. He was sure his son had appendicitis and brought him to the emergency room. The surgeon who was supposed to do the job was reluctant, maybe in part because he didn't want to get it wrong for the family member of another physician. My friend, who is an orthopedic surgeon, felt the appendix needed to come out. So he told the surgeon who needed to get going, "I want to pay you to take out my son's normal appendix!" They struck a deal, and the appendix was removed (which was verified later to be infected).

I had to smile when I got the final report back from the pathologist regarding my own patient from that 4th of July. It did show appendicitis. Sam had probably had a mild attack each of the prior times. The dad had made the right call to get the job done once and for all.

# Incidental Miracles

My friend and colleague, a surgeon, caught me in the hall. He had a small lump on his posterior that he wanted removed. I was free and we walked down to the ambulatory surgery area. The nurse was available and didn't mind. She helped to set up.

He had a lump that appeared to be about half the size of my thumb. This would typically be a little fatty tumor, called a *lipoma*. It shouldn't be a big deal to numb up and remove.

As we got going, it appeared that it was bigger than expected. In fact, as I continued on, it appeared that it was going be approximately the size of my fist. The nurse didn't want to get involved assisting in removing something this size and became more and more scarce. I kept checking with my buddy to see if we should stop, stitch it up, and try again some other time in the operating room.

He said, "I'm doing okay. Keep on going."

I kept adding a little more of the numbing medicine and we kept on going.

All of a sudden he jumped (it seemed like about a foot in the air to me).

"Yeuow!"

"Are you okay?"

"Yeah. I am now. I guess just keep on going."

We finished and I stitched him up uneventfully.

He lived near me and I went to visit him about a week later. He was down on his hands and knees doing slot cars in his living room.

"What the heck? What are you doing?"

"I haven't been able to do slot cars for years. Since school. Whatever you cut that day cured me."

He went on to tell me how he had pursued a cure for his back pain for years. He had seen medical doctors, surgeons, chiropractors, and acupuncture physicians. He had multiple x-rays and scans and tests. He had had multiple therapies, even including acupuncture to his testicles. Nothing had made any difference for his back pain until I removed his "lipoma."

I apparently had cut some nerve that this otherwise unremarkable benign tumor of fat was lying against. He couldn't adequately express his gratitude for the cure of this chronic problem.

*****

I see many people in my practice with "chronic abdominal pain issues." Often they've seen multiple doctors and therapists over the years and they've had many different treatments performed. They're hopeful that an operation will take care of their problem. I typically have a conversation with them, pointing out that there's a potential long list of problems that may be causing their pain. I may be able to help them by targeting one or two of the potential sources on the list, but there are certainly no guarantees. My general observation is that if two or three reasonably smart physicians don't figure out this type of problem, the odds of the next physician figuring it out spiral down rapidly. Just as in the case of my friend, I note that many times people go on searching for years until they get the one hint that will help them solve their problem. As anticipated, it seems like nothing short of a miracle in those few instances when you do trip across the source of their chronic pain and fix it.

One such person was a healthy woman in her 50s who came in with a hernia in the right groin. We scheduled her repair, which would be straightforward. She commented that she had been experiencing an increasing pain up under her left ribs. I told her that I didn't think the hernia repair would affect it. This is what she had anticipated I would say.

When I went in to fix the hernia, it turned out she had fatty tissue from the left upper abdomen that was caught in the hernia. I fixed it, not thinking much of the finding at the time. To my surprise, she told me on her return visit several weeks later that the pain in her left upper abdomen was gone for the first time in years. Those unanticipated blessings from surgery can be like a gift – both to the patient and the surgeon.

---

*One time we came in to pick up the patient and he was gone. The IV was hanging from the pole on his bed. His wife caught him at the front door leaving with his hospital gown "aflappin." She "took him by the ear" and brought him back to surgery. He was a 45-year-old executive. He had a panic attack and had hit the road. So now I often say to patients waiting for surgery, "Don't run away now!"*

# Hits and Heroics

Once or twice a year my partners and I become "ships passing in the night." This would be one of those days.

I had to leave for a non-negotiable meeting at noon on Thursday. My partner was covering the call for me until Friday morning. But he was leaving town Friday morning, so I would take over call for the day on Friday. Then our other associate would take over call on Friday evening for the weekend.

Normally this should not be too difficult. But it happened that I already had a full day scheduled on Friday that would start with office in the morning to be followed with two cases of surgery in the afternoon.

On Thursday afternoon, my partner added a case to my schedule on Friday. His Thursday afternoon patient, Ernie, needed a portacath for chemotherapy. He did not want to wait without eating and requested a better spot on Friday. So I had added him onto the schedule to be done "quickly" before the office opened on Friday morning.

My first sense of storm clouds on the horizon came when I received an 11:30 PM phone call on Thursday evening from the emergency room. Normally my phone would have been turned off since I was not yet on call, but it had stayed on for some reason. I told the emergency room that it was my partner who was on call. I called the service to make sure they had this noted correctly. All this was not a big deal, except for the fact that I now knew something was brewing in the emergency room. There was a good chance I'd get to deal with it in the morning, after my partner had left.

So I got up early to be there in time to sort out the issues. Sure enough, there were two people who needed evaluation for appendicitis, for which surgery was a possible outcome. And before I could get up from my seat from checking in, I received a call for a third appendix. Normally we do an appendix as soon as possible when we find out about it. I knew I would have to do a little hustling to figure out how to fit all this in.

So I began my triage. One appendix, Roxanne, needed to go right away. I postponed the previously arranged surgery and booked this case. The second appendix was a false alarm and was eventually discharged. The third appendix was Donna, a 37 weeks pregnant woman. She was pretty comfortable, so she could wait until after the office. Not ideal, but doable. The man who didn't want to wait yesterday so he could eat would have to wait today. It figures.

So by 6:20 AM I had figured out I needed to switch the order and do the appendix first. I called the operating room to start arrangements. The person running the desk didn't seem very excited about this. He said there was no staff. I told him I had walked in with the crew so I presumed things could get underway fairly quickly. I told him that I thought it would be reasonable to start at 6:45 AM. He didn't seem excited about this either, but he said he would start the arrangements. I did my best to make my intent as clear as possible for the sake of the patients, me, and the OR staff.

I continued to triage in the meantime (walking through the ER and evaluating the patients). I checked in with the OR about 6:45 AM to see if we could get going. Roxanne had arrived in the holding area, but nothing else seemed to be getting done. I checked back at 7 AM, and there was still no action. I asked the nurse for help and she started to get things rolling. Anesthesia changed positions several times (because the person on from night before doesn't want to start the case and wants the new person coming in to take it) but finally completed their check-in (a series of steps they need to complete to prepare the patient).

The people in the operating room responsible for setting up were starting their work as well. Some days (and some people) make surgery feel like it takes 42,000 steps. Other times it seems like it flows with about four steps (consent, anesthesia, prep, scalpel). This day was unfolding like a 42,000 step day.

Due to the delay, I then needed to decide if I would continue on with Roxanne's surgery and be late to the office, or postpone the case and be on time. My 25 minutes of prep time had turned into 55 minutes of prep time. Office started at eight. I figured I would still give it a shot.

After everyone had finished their checking-in work, I started to roll the patient, Roxanne, down the hall. It's not often that I did this and I raised a few eyebrows. The nurses continued to set up in the room. We had at least 20 minutes of further preparation to do, including putting the patient to sleep etc. It seemed to me that the nurses had plenty of time for their set up as well.

I'm not sure they agreed, because one of the nurses said, "This is disrespectful." What she meant, of course, was that I was showing a lack of respect for their wanting to do their jobs properly by making them go faster than they wanted to.

"What did you say?" I turned to the nurse, who was a highly competent colleague.

Meanwhile, as Roxanne was getting on the operating room table, I could see her eyes getting bigger and bigger.

"I said I think this is disrespectful to the patient."

Ouch. After everything I had done to help everyone get the patient ready, I felt like Rodney Dangerfield ("I don't get no respect…"). I took a short walk to regain my composure and returned back to my room. Ironically, on days like this, it helps me to refer to it as the "happy room."

I personally have a blind spot the size of Texas regarding a response in these situations. My spiritual journey lately has been lessons in how to respond in any situation from the place of love within myself. In a perfect, controlled situation (I wish!), I could reflect before acting: *How would responding in love look for the OR staff, the patient, myself? Would this add to the vulnerability of everyone involved or simply solve the issues?* I have certainly noticed over the years that people I respect who are "higher on the feeding chain" seem to lose their temper a lot less than the average Joe. So I'm aware that in addition to demonstrating my skill as a surgeon, every situation is also an opportunity to improve my self control and allow "love" to be present.

That said, I still find it a huge challenge to practice a "loving" response when there is a shortage of time and resources. I pushed this case through the OR, although I still believe I did the right thing. I also realize my actions created ill will between myself and my colleague.

The nurse and I didn't say much more that day. I finished the case and I was 25 minutes late to the office, but no worse for the wear. Roxanne did need her appendix removed, and I was glad to have accomplished it.

As soon as the office work was completed, we prepared to do the appendectomy on the other woman, Donna, who was 37 weeks pregnant. This was a little tricky, because normally we wouldn't attempt a laparoscopic surgery on someone who is more than 20 weeks pregnant. There would not be much room for me to work inside the abdomen. The anesthesiologist expressed concern about this several times. I responded that all we could do was try.

In the end, when it was all said and done, this surgery was not very hard. I was pretty happy that we completed it without any problems. We finished the rest of the cases. My man, Ernie, who wanted to eat, ended up going into surgery at about 6:00 in the evening. I was glad that he persevered and hung around, or we might not have completed it until Monday with the weekend coming. We finished about 8 PM, so I was able to finish the rest of the office paperwork by about 10 PM.

*Michael DeHaan*

*****

I was gone the weekend following this Friday. I came back on Monday morning and checked on the patients. Donna, the pregnant woman with the appendectomy, was sitting in a chair smiling with a new baby. I laughed, delighted that she had delivered. In fact, her water had broken on the way back from surgery to her room. Fortunately, she had a veteran obstetrician and she went on to deliver uneventfully. It was a perfect ending to my "difficult" appendectomy on the 37 week pregnancy.

The same obstetrician had once helped take out a larger rectal cancer behind a uterus in a 20 week pregnancy. The university doctors weren't willing to tackle the case without aborting the baby first. The patient refused this, and ended up with us. So he held the uterus and fetus up while I completed the surgery.

Never a dull moment. I'm thankful that even with the sometimes frustrating dynamics of the operating room, we remember that taking care of the patient is our first priority.

---

*A reminder for surgeons: When you stop the elevator door from closing, it's recommended that you stick your head in the door and not your hands. You don't want to risk damaging a critical body part.*

## Not tonight, Frank

She wasn't in the mood.

It was a slow day on the service. I was in my third year of surgical residency. We were working for the busiest surgeon at our hospital. He normally would be doing some big difficult case. Instead, we were taking the opportunity to walk around and see each patient. We were excited because we didn't get the chance to do this very often.

There were almost 20 of us total. Chief resident, Junior residents, medical students, and various other people. At each room we would have a discussion about the topic that each patient presented. It was occasionally a little uncomfortable because a question would typically be targeted just a little above your current level of ability. This could leave you a little embarrassed at times. You would really remember the answer, however, once you got it. In any case, the process generally served as an excellent teaching tool.

It was a fairly dignified entourage. We were seeing people who were sick and it generally didn't afford any levity. In addition, we were each concerned that we would get caught on a question for which we didn't know the answer. It kept you on your toes.

The woman in the next room was elderly and had come from the nursing home. She had a bed sore on her back just above her behind. Overall, not a big surgical issue. Still, it generated the usual discussion on the science of the problem. Prolonged pressure on any spot can cause *ischemia* (loss of blood supply). Within hours, tissue breakdown can begin. The problem is most often related to a host of other problems that are playing out. The most difficult part, however, is that typically these ulcers are the sign of a failing person. It is possible to successfully manage an ulcer, but it's often difficult to change the course of someone who is generally failing..

In any case, we were ready to go see the patient and view her ulceration. We filed into the room and gathered around her bed, introducing ourselves as necessary to help her understand the group. The senior surgeon asked several of us to roll her over gently so that we could view her problem. Simultaneously with our movement to pull her over, there was a brief but distinct pause in the conversation. In the quiet of the room, we could all hear her quietly request, "Not tonight, Frank."

It started with soft smiles around the room, but eventually we couldn't hold back the snickers. We politely thanked her for the visit and excused ourselves from the room. We had a good chuckle, and in the end we had to quit our rounds. It was a little hard not to feel that a poignant detail of her life had been revealed before our eyes.

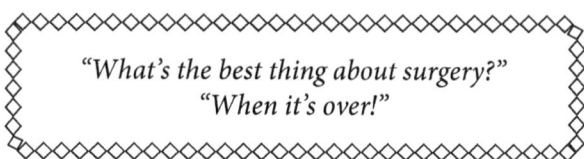

*"What's the best thing about surgery?"*
*"When it's over!"*

# Epilogue

My work as a surgeon has put me in touch with people in the most intimate, personal way. It is often an amazing experience to play an integral role in a person's healing journey. For some patients, an encounter with their surgeon may be one of the most memorable events of their life, especially if cancer or permanent alternation in their body is involved.

My experience with surgery has provided a unique window to life in general. As a surgeon, I employ my skill to create an environment for healing to take place. Even when all has been executed to perfection, why do some patients get to live and some don't? The science of it draws one away from spirituality, but the humanity of it draws one closer. All together, it's changed my spiritual journey and I feel like it's added to my perception of the Grand Intelligence.

My preacher says that young people sometimes ask, "What job should I be doing to further my spiritual growth?" But perhaps, as Jesus said, we are asking the wrong question. Maybe the question is, "How can whatever job I choose help me to grow spiritually?" In some way for all of us, work is a vehicle for our spiritual expansion, both in the opportunity for personal accomplishment and in the learning that comes through relationship with others.

In some ways, these are everyday stories about feelings and issues we all struggle with, regardless of the work we do. I hope you enjoyed reading these stories as much as I enjoyed writing them.

Send comments to:

handsandheart59@gmail.com

www.ingramcontent.com/pod-product-compliance
Ingram Content Group UK Ltd.
Pitfield, Milton Keynes, MK11 3LW, UK
UKHW041946230426
12048UKWH00008B/159